Discontinuing Antidepressant Medications

Discontinuing Antidepressant Medications

GIOVANNI A. FAVA

Clinical Professor of Psychiatry, University at Buffalo,
State University of New York, Buffalo, New York, USA

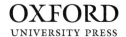
OXFORD
UNIVERSITY PRESS

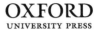

Great Clarendon Street, Oxford, OX2 6DP,
United Kingdom

Oxford University Press is a department of the University of Oxford.
It furthers the University's objective of excellence in research, scholarship,
and education by publishing worldwide. Oxford is a registered trade mark of
Oxford University Press in the UK and in certain other countries

First Edition published in 2021

Impression: 1

Published in the United States of America by Oxford University Press
198 Madison Avenue, New York, NY 10016, United States of America

British Library Cataloguing in Publication Data

Data available

Library of Congress Control Number: 2021945152

ISBN 978–0–19–289664–3

DOI: 10.1093/med/9780192896643.001.0001

Printed and bound by
CPI Group (UK) Ltd, Croydon, CR0 4YY

Preface

The clinical problems that may ensue when antidepressant medications are discontinued have been neglected by the scientific literature. Patients experiencing the anguish and mental pain of withdrawal syndromes have not received appropriate medical attention and have been forced to refer themselves to websites, groups, and associations, which have the recognized merit of providing support but cannot offer the medical competence required. This book attempts to fill this gap. It provides a detailed account of assessment and management strategies, drawing from the literature that is available and the extensive personal experience of the author.

The author is indebted to the members of the Affective Disorders Program where most of his clinical experience originated: Nicoletta Sonino (consultant for internal medicine and endocrinology); Chiara Rafanelli and Anna Rita Raffi (consultants for psychiatry and psychotherapy); and Carlotta Belaise, Jenny Guidi, Laura Staccini, and Elena Tomba (consultants for psychology and psychotherapy). In particular, Jenny Guidi, Fiammetta Cosci, and Nicoletta Sonino gave important suggestions and feedback. Another essential contribution came from Guy Chouinard, who provided important sources of insight. The author is also grateful to Giada Benasi, Danilo Carrozzino, Marcella Lucente, Emanuela Offidani, and Chiara Patierno for their help and support.

Contents

Abbreviations

BZ	benzodiazepine
CBT	cognitive-behavioral therapy
DCPR	Diagnostic Criteria for Psychosomatic Research
DESS	Discontinuation-Emergent Signs and Symptoms (questionnaire)
DSM	Diagnostic and Statistical Manual of Mental Disorders
EBM	evidence-based medicine
FDA	Food and Drug Administration
MAO	monoamine oxidase
MBE	medicine-based evidence
MPQ	Mental Pain Questionnaire
PSSD	post-SSRI sexual dysfunction
PTSD	post-traumatic stress disorder
RCT	randomized controlled trial
SNRI	serotonin-noradrenaline reuptake inhibitor
SSRI	selective serotonin reuptake inhibitor
STAR*D	Sequenced Treatment Alternatives to Relieve Depression
TCA	tricyclic antidepressant
WBT	Well-Being Therapy

1
Gaining Insight of the Problem

When I started my residency training program in psychiatry in Italy, more than four decades ago, depression was the psychiatric disorder that particularly attracted my attention. In 1980, I decided to move to the United States to further pursue my interest, first in Albuquerque, New Mexico, and then in Buffalo, New York, where I was invited to establish a depression unit. I was convinced that depression was essentially an episodic disorder, that there were powerful remedies against it (antidepressant drugs), and that chronicity was essentially a consequence of inadequate diagnosis and treatment. Today, if I think of my views then, I am surprised by my naiveté and clinical blindness, although such views were shared by almost every expert in the field. We have since become aware that depression is essentially a chronic disorder with multiple acute episodes along its course (1).

While working in the United States, I had essentially a cross-sectional view of the disorder (I was assessing patients while they were in the hospital, and I had no clue as to what happened after their discharge). However when, in the late eighties, I decided to go back to Italy and to establish an outpatient clinic at the University of Bologna with opportunities for follow-up, things looked quite different. Also, patients I had personally treated with antidepressant drugs and whom I had judged to have completely remitted relapsed into depression after some time. What was I missing?

In the meanwhile, an increasing number of studies were pointing to the fact that the pharmacological treatment of depression was not solving all the problems and, despite substantial improvement, important residual symptoms remained (2). Such symptoms particularly included anxiety and irritability, and were associated with impaired functional capacity. Most residual symptoms were present also in the prodromal phase of illness and might progress to become prodromal symptoms of relapse

(2). In the nineties, I thus devised a treatment strategy that departed from current approaches: the sequential model (3). It was an intensive, two-stage approach, where one type of treatment (psychotherapy) was employed to improve symptoms which another type of treatment (pharmacotherapy) was unable to affect. The rationale of this approach was to use psychotherapeutic strategies when they are most likely to make a unique and distinct contribution to patient well-being and to achieve a more complete recovery by addressing residual symptomatology (3). The sequential design was different from maintenance strategies for prolonging clinical responses that therapies of the acute episodes have obtained, as well as from augmentation or switching strategies, because of the lack of response to the first line of treatment.

In the nineties, I designed and conducted two randomized controlled trials (RCTs) concerned with the sequential model of treatment of depression: pharmacotherapy of the acute episode followed by a modified form of cognitive behavioral therapy compared to clinical management (the same amount of time is spent with the patient, but without specific interventions or homework assignments), while antidepressant drugs were tapered and discontinued (4, 5). The drugs that were used were mostly tricyclic antidepressants (TCAs). Withdrawal symptoms following discontinuation were soon recognized after the introduction of TCAs (6), and I was thus aware that they could ensue during tapering or after discontinuation of the medications (7). Based on my clinical experience, I had devised the following protocol: antidepressants were tapered at the slowest possible rate every other week. For instance, if a patient had achieved remission with the use of 150 mg of amitriptyline, the medication was tapered at the rate of 25 mg every other week, until discontinuation. I also provided one session of psychotherapy every two weeks, during which I could monitor discontinuation. I personally treated all 88 patients who entered the trials (4, 5); only in eight cases was tapering stopped due to the re-emergence of depressed mood (for six patients, tapering was successful a few months later outside of these studies). I had alerted the patients to call me if they perceived any "steps" (a qualitative difference from the psychological state of the previous dosage). In no cases were withdrawal symptoms observed. In those days, it thus appeared that antidepressant drugs were unlikely to induce dependence and withdrawal symptoms upon tapering and discontinuation.

In another study that I conducted in that period (8), 20 patients with panic disorder and agoraphobia, who had been successfully treated with a standardized behavioral protocol and were taking benzodiazepines (BZs), had their medications gradually tapered and discontinued. The design of the study was to analyze withdrawal symptoms in a setting not contaminated by the re-emergence of the anxiety disorder. Successful discontinuation was achieved in 16 patients, but 13 suffered from withdrawal symptoms. Discontinuation was not feasible in an additional four patients. It was clear to me then that TCAs and BZs were quite different in their dependence potential.

The Emergence of Second-Generation Antidepressants

In the nineties, however, quite a different picture emerged with the introduction of selective serotonin reuptake inhibitors (SSRIs). We started being confronted with the withdrawal syndromes that ensued with their tapering and discontinuation. My first experience was a wake-up call (9).

Alan was a 43-year-old executive with a 4-month history of a major depressive episode who had been treated by his primary care physician with paroxetine 40 mg/day. He had displayed only a partial response to the medication and was thus referred to me "for something stronger." Indeed, I thought that a TCA, desipramine, could obtain better results. I reduced paroxetine to 20 mg and, after 3 days, I switched it to desipramine, with an initial dosage of 50 mg/day. After a week of desipramine treatment (increased to 100 mg/day), Alan called me up and asked me to see him urgently. He did not want to anticipate anything on the phone, but I perceived he was extremely worried. He just said "I cannot make it another night this way." I was able to see him the very same day. He had experienced severe vertigo, gait instability, malaise, muscle aches, and hypnagogic visual hallucinations (geometrical designs, abstract shapes, or scenes as from movies on falling asleep). Alan was terrified. "What is going on here?" he asked me. I had the feeling of something truly organic. Alan denied using other medications or recreational drugs, and I felt I could trust him. I wondered about a medical disease, but there was no fever or other signs. I performed a physical examination, but that was totally negative. I thus tried to reassure him, saying that these were temporary side effects due to the rapid medication change. Desipramine was decreased to 25 mg/day and, in 3 days, it was discontinued. I wanted the patient to be off any medications. It took 10 (long) days for the new symptoms to fade. At that point, I started desipramine again, which I progressively and slowly increased to 150 mg/day. Alan fully responded after 4 weeks and all withdrawal symptoms disappeared.

As Alan, I also wondered what went on. I looked into the literature and I found two letters documenting similar, though less violent, withdrawal symptoms after paroxetine discontinuation (10, 11). In a patient described in one of these reports (11), the addition of fluoxetine stopped the withdrawal effects of paroxetine, suggesting that the syndrome could be serotonergically mediated. Dilsaver (7) postulated that withdrawal phenomena could be mediated by cholinergic mechanisms, which in the case of Alan, however, were excluded since desipramine and paroxetine bind to the muscarinic cholinergic receptor with approximately equal affinity (12).

After Alan's case, I thought that I should be more cautious in tapering SSRIs, using the methods that I had applied to TCAs in the studies on sequential treatment—that is, the smallest decrement possible every other week (4, 5). Nonetheless, despite these precautions, withdrawal symptoms ensued with all types of SSRI, even though this did not happen all the time. There was an upsurge of case reports in the literature, followed by double-blind controlled investigations, that alerted the clinician to the potential occurrence of withdrawal syndromes upon discontinuation of SSRIs and also serotonin-noradrenaline reuptake inhibitors (SNRIs) such as venlafaxine, as summarized by several reviews that were published (13–17).

However, in the nineties and the first decade of the new millennium, the pharmaceutical industry urged the downplaying of withdrawal manifestations upon discontinuation of SSRIs and SNRIs. The commercial plan was to expand the use of SSRIs and SNRIs from depression to other psychiatric disorders (particularly anxiety disturbances) and to prolong their administration to the longest possible time. Awareness of the occurrence of dependence would have run counter to such a strategy. Withdrawal reactions were promptly renamed as discontinuation syndromes, as if they were different from other psychotropic drugs such as

BZs (even though there was no evidence to support that dependence was different). Both physicians and patients were taught that the problem manifests itself only with abrupt discontinuation of antidepressant medications and that, if symptoms arise, they have to be considered signs of relapse, with prompt re-administration of the antidepressant.

Many clinicians, in all specialties and types of practice, were able to perceive there was something wrong with the approach dictated by the pharmaceutical industry and its prodigal experts. However, I suspect they were reluctant to voice that the emperor had no clothes because the scientific literature was consistent, with very few exceptions, in praising the emperor's clothes.

The Insights of a Clinical Investigation

With my colleague Chiara Rafanelli, we designed a study that was similar to the one that was employed with BZ discontinuation (8) for testing the feasibility of getting patients with panic disorder and agoraphobia off SSRIs. Again, I personally treated all patients. Twenty subjects who had been successfully treated with a standardized behavioral protocol based on exposure homework and were taking SSRIs had their medications gradually tapered and discontinued (18). We thought we had the best possible conditions for discontinuing SSRIs: patients were panic-free after a type of psychotherapy that was associated with enduring effects (19), and they received individual attention, with opportunities for clarification and discussion of any symptoms that might have appeared. I managed both psychotherapy and pharmacotherapy. Yet the results were disappointing. Nine of the patients (45%) experienced a withdrawal syndrome, which subsided within a month in all but three patients who had been taking paroxetine (18). These three patients developed cyclothymia, which they had never experienced before, and presented with a syndrome that was later defined as persistent postwithdrawal disorder (20)—that is, the protraction of withdrawal symptomatology and/or return of original symptoms at greater intensity and/or with additional symptoms related to an emerging new mental disorder. They were all treated with clonazepam: in one case, the response was good; in another, it was very limited and symptoms subsided when paroxetine was administered again; and in the third, clonazepam yielded no improvement, and the symptoms went on for 3 years before fading (with the patient refusing to take paroxetine again). Nothing like this had happened with BZs: indeed, anxiety improved upon discontinuation (8), in line with published literature (21).

Our results were in sharp contrast with what was preached by key opinion leaders. In my experience, withdrawal symptoms could occur also with very slow tapering in remitted patients; in almost half of patients, disturbances were severe and disabling, and did not necessarily fade away in 2–3 weeks. It was thus clear how so many patients were struggling with discontinuing antidepressant medications. If things were difficult in those conditions, how would they be for a person trying to find a way out by himself/herself? A few patients in the study confided that without me (someone they trusted to help them get rid of their agoraphobia) to explain the temporary nature of the phenomena, they would have given up their attempts to stop medication. Yet, ours was only a brief report in a psychopharmacology journal in 2007 (18). How could we compete with massive propaganda, reviews in mainstream journals, lectures, and symposia at meetings?

Our findings on the persistence of withdrawal symptoms, with the potential addition of new clinical phenomena, had been anticipated by Guy Chouinard's group in Montreal (22). A few months after our paper had appeared (18), he wrote to inform me that he was going to be in Italy and would like to meet me. I thought this was a fantastic opportunity: I was a great admirer of his groundbreaking work as a clinical pharmacologist (he had introduced the clinical use of so many psychotropic drugs, including fluoxetine and clonazepam) and of his creativity, methodological rigor, and intellectual honesty. He was staying in Parma, not far from Bologna. I took a train. He was waiting for me at the train station. We found a café nearby and spent about an hour sharing our views. What a comfort it was to hear that I was not alone in advancing certain hypotheses about SSRI and SNRI withdrawal phenomena. Regrettably, I soon had to catch the train back, but we started a collaboration and a friendship that was essential for the developments of the following years. I was lucky to be able to take advantage of his frequent visits to Italy. Going back to Bologna that evening in the train, I repeated what my patient Alan had asked me: "What is going on here?" I felt we had the moral and intellectual obligation to provide an answer, no matter what the personal costs might be.

I was fully aware how the battle was going to be. Twenty years ago, the journal I edit, *Psychotherapy and Psychosomatics*, anticipated the current medical scenario dominated by corporate interests which result in self-selected academic oligarchies (special interest groups) that influence clinical and scientific information (23). Members of special interest groups, by virtue of their financial power and close ties among themselves, systematically prevent dissemination of data which may be in conflict with their interests. Corporate powers have fused with academic medicine to create an unhealthy alliance that works against objective reporting of clinical research, that sets up meetings and symposia with the specific purpose of selling the participants to sponsors, and that substantially controls journals, medical associations, and related foundations (through direct support and/or advertising) (24). Such phenomena operate in all branches of medicine, including psychiatry (25). We were only a group of scattered people behind a small, independent journal, questioning the current views and building a counterculture, but I was determined to accept the challenge.

References

1. Fava GA, Tomba E, Grandi S: The road to recovery from depression. Psychother Psychosom 2007; 76:260–5.
2. Fava GA, Kellner R: Prodromal symptoms in affective disorders. Am J Psychiatry 1991; 148:823–30.
3. Fava GA: Sequential treatment: a new way of integrating pharmacotherapy and psychotherapy. Psychother Psychosom 1999; 68:227–9.
4. Fava GA, Grandi S, Zielezny M, Canestrari R, Morphy MA: Cognitive behavioral treatment of residual symptoms in primary major depressive disorder. Am J Psychiatry 1994; 151:1295–9.
5. Fava GA, Rafanelli C, Grandi S, Conti S, Belluardo P: Prevention of recurrent depression with cognitive behavioral therapy. Arch Gen Psychiatry 1998; 55:816–20.
6. Kramer JC, Klein DF, Fink M: Withdrawal symptoms following discontinuation of imipramine therapy. Am J Psychiatry 1961; 118:549–50.
7. Dilsaver SC: Heterocyclic antidepressant, monoamine oxidase inhibitor and neuroleptic withdrawal phenomena. Prog Neuro-psychopharmacol Biol Psychiatry 1990; 14:137–61.
8. Fava GA, Grandi S, Belluardo P, Savron G, Raffi AR, Conti S, Saviotti FM: Benzodiazepines and anxiety sensitivity in panic disorder. Prog Neuro-psychopharmacol Biol Psychiatry 1994; 18:1163–8.

9. Fava GA, Grandi S: Withdrawal syndromes after paroxetine and sertraline discontinuation. J Clin Psychopharmacol 1995; 15:374–5.

10. Barr LC, Goodman WK, Price LH: Physical symptoms associated with paroxetine discontinuation. Am J Psychiatry 1994; 151:289.

11. Keuthen NG, Cyr P, Ricciardi JA, Minichiello WE, Buttolph ML, Jenike MA: Medication withdrawal symptoms in obsessive-compulsive disorder patients treated with paroxetine. J Clin Psychopharmacol 1994; 14:206–7.

12. Thomas DR, Nelson DR, Johnson AM. Biochemical effects of the antidepressant paroxetine, a specific 5-hydroxytryptamine uptake inhibitor. Psychopharmacology 1987; 93:193–200.

13. Lojoyeux M, Ades J: Antidepressant discontinuation. J Clin Psychiatry 1997; 58 (suppl.7):11–16.

14. Zajecka J, Tracy KA, Mitchell, S: Discontinuation symptoms after treatment with serotonin reuptake inhibitors. J Clin Psychiatry 1997; 58:291–7.

15. Haddad PM: Antidepressant discontinuation syndromes. Drug Safety 2001; 24:183–97.

16. Schatzberg AF, Blier P, Delgado PL, Fava M, Haddad PM, Shelton RC: Antidepressant discontinuation syndrome. J Clin Psychiatry 2006; 67 (suppl.4):27–30.

17. Warner CH, Bobo W, Warner C, Reid S, Rachal J: Antidepressant discontinuation syndrome. Am Fam Physician 2006; 74:449–56.

18. Fava GA, Bernardi M, Tomba E, Rafanelli C: Effects of gradual discontinuation of selective serotonin reuptake inhibitors in panic disorder with agoraphobia. Int J Neuropsychopharmacol 2007; 10:835–8.

19. Fava GA, Rafanelli C, Grandi S, Conti S, Ruini C, Mangelli L, Belluardo P: Long-term outcome of panic disorder with agoraphobia treated by exposure. Psychol Med 2001; 31:891–8.

20. Chouinard G, Chouinard VA: New classification of selective serotonin reuptake inhibitor withdrawal. Psychother Psychosom 2015; 84:63–71.

21. Rickels K, Schweizer E, Case G, Greenblatt DJ: Long-term therapeutic use of benzodiazepines: I. Effects of abrupt discontinuation. Arch Gen Psychiatry 1990; 47:899–907.

22. Bhanji N, Chouinard G, Kolivakis T, Margolese H: Persistent tardive rebound panic disorder, rebound anxiety and insomnia following paroxetine withdrawal: a review of rebound withdrawal phenomena. Can J Clin Pharmacol 2006; 13:69–74.

23. Fava GA: Conflict of interest and special interest groups. Psychother Psychosom 2001; 70:1–5.

24. Fava GA: The hidden costs of financial conflicts of interest in medicine. Psychother Psychosom 2016; 85:65–70.

25. Whitaker R, Cosgrove L: Psychiatry Under the Influence. New York, Palgrave MacMillan, 2015.

2

The Clinical Manifestations of Withdrawal Following Discontinuation of Antidepressant Drugs

After the first reports in the mid-nineties on withdrawal syndromes from antidepressants, there was an upsurge of investigations, reviews, and symposia on the topic in the following decade. Such a phase was then followed by a clear-cut decrease in interest, as if the "epidemic" was no longer of public concern. The pharmaceutical industry had been quite successful in minimizing these clinical events and probably opted for discussing these matters as little as possible.

Another phenomenon was, however, on the rise. In 1998, I had received a letter from Charles Medawar, the director of a consumers association in the UK, the Social Audit. He had opened a website for hosting reports from the people on their reactions to SSRIs withdrawal and had published an account of these shared experiences (1). Other websites followed including, in particular, one initiated by Adele Framer in the USA (under the pseudonym of Altostrata) (http://survivingantidepressants. org), offering tapering information and peer support for withdrawal and protracted withdrawal syndromes from psychiatric drugs. Another, initiated by Robert Whitaker (http://madinamerica.com), provided an important point of encounter for patients and clinicians for discussing issues that were censored by mainstream psychiatry.

In 2002, I received (and published in *Psychotherapy and Psychosomatics*) a letter by a young psychologist sharing his experience with discontinuing paroxetine: "Starting the medication was easy. After a particularly rough breakup with a girlfriend who had left me very upset and listless for a few weeks, my psychiatrist prescribed 20 mg of paroxetine. Taking the medication became part of my daily life" (2, p. 237). When he decided to stop the medication (with an intermediate step at 10 mg), a different story emerged. It was a nightmare of agitation, irritability, and physical sensations such as "zaps"—experiences described as "feeling of electricity that would start with a blurring dizziness and then washed over my entire body" (2, p. 237). The withdrawal experience lasted 4 weeks and the letter closed with the recommendation of informing patients about these problems before prescribing a SSRIs, for an informed choice.

I admired the courage of this young psychologist in sharing his experience. Guy Chouinard decided to explore—with the help of a gifted clinical psychologist from my team, Carlotta Belaise, and his daughter, Virginie-Anne, a psychiatrist—the websites that were concerned with withdrawal reactions from antidepressant drugs (3). Despite the obvious limitations of these sources (e.g., subjects might also have taken other drugs, clinical assessments were not available), they found that the symptoms confirmed those reported by the literature, and that the manifestations and duration of symptoms could be very different from one patient to another. They also observed that the persistent postwithdrawal disorders we had reported (4, 5) appeared to be quite common. Such findings were confirmed by a recent report (6), which outlined the lack of information given to the patient, the inability to diagnose and treat withdrawal syndromes, and the resulting tendency of patients to seek advice outside of healthcare, including from online forums.

A major consequence of the neglect of professional organizations and scientific societies to ensure proper care to people has been that patients experiencing the anguish and mental pain of withdrawal syndromes are unlikely to receive appropriate medical attention and are forced to refer themselves to websites, groups, and associations, which have the recognized merit of providing support but are unable to offer the medical competence that is required.

We attempted to provide some medical help and competence. I was struck by the fact that the reviews that were available were characterized by a selective use of the literature, with a strong commercial bias (and indeed most of the authors had major financial conflicts of interest). With the help of a number of members of our research group (particularly

Carlotta Belaise, Jenny Guidi, Emanuela Offidani, Giada Benasi, and Marcella Lucente), I thought it was important to perform two systematic reviews (one about SSRIs, the other about SNRIs) of the relevant literature. The term "systematic" implies that we attempted to trace and consider all the papers (including case reports) that appeared in the scientific literature and were indexed in such major databases as PubMed. Of course systematic reviews are also, in the end, subjective, because of the nature of the synthesis and interpretation, which may amplify some aspects and neglect other issues. Systematic reviews are also very liable to the presence of financial conflicts of interest and often lack the presence of an author with clinical familiarity with the topic (7). Our lack of financial conflicts of interests and our clinical work were the basis of our syntheses and interpretations. Not surprisingly, our papers took two years to be completed.

Guy Chouinard dedicated himself to the development of diagnostic criteria that could facilitate the recognition of clinical phenomena related to withdrawal. He was supported by another member of our research network, Fiammetta Cosci, who contributed to several important aspects.

Findings of Systematic Reviews on the Clinical Manifestations of Withdrawal

In 2015, we published our systematic review on withdrawal symptoms after SSRIs (paroxetine, fluoxetine, sertraline, fluvoxamine, citalopram, escitalopram) tapering and/or discontinuation (8). In 2018, our systematic review on SNRIs (duloxetine, venlafaxine, desvenlafaxine, milnacipran, levomilnacipran) was released (9). Hengartner et al. (10) remarked that these were the first systematic reviews and appeared after nearly two hundred meta-analyses on the efficacy of new-generation antidepressants. The results of the two reviews were pretty similar and are summarized here:

1. Withdrawal symptoms occurred with any SSRIs and SNRIs. However, in controlled trials, paroxetine and venlafaxine had significantly higher prevalence rates compared to other antidepressants. The prevalence of withdrawal syndromes varied also across

studies and its correct estimation was hindered by a lack of case identification in many instances.

2. Gradual tapering did not eliminate the risk of withdrawal reactions. Indeed, a significant advantage of gradual tapering compared to abrupt discontinuation did not emerge, with SSRIs or SNRIs.

3. Withdrawal symptoms included a wide range of clinical manifestations (Box 2.1), and were similar after the discontinuation of SSRIs or SNRIs. The withdrawal syndrome encompassed a broad range of somatic symptoms (e.g., headache, dizziness, flu-like symptoms, nausea). Psychological symptoms such as agitation, anxiety, panic attacks, dysphoria, irritability, confusion, and worsening of mood occurred as well. Symptoms typically began within 3 days of stopping antidepressant medication or initiating medication taper. Untreated symptoms could be mild and resolve spontaneously in 1–3 weeks; in other cases, however, they persisted for months or even years, suggesting the presence of persistent postwithdrawal disorders.

4. SSRIs and SNRIs should be added to the list of drugs potentially inducing dependence and withdrawal phenomena. The findings should caution the physician to prescribe them in the setting of chronic pain, as it particularly applies to duloxetine.

5. The term "discontinuation syndrome" minimizes the vulnerabilities induced by SSRIs and SNRIs and should be replaced by "withdrawal syndrome."

In 2020, Cosci and Chouinard provided an overview of acute and persistent withdrawal syndromes following discontinuation of psychotropic medications (11). The following conclusions were reached:

1. In addition to TCAs, monoamine oxidase (MAO) inhibitors, SSRIs, and SNRIs, withdrawal syndromes were reported with any other antidepressant. When no specific literature was found (i.e., vilazodone and vortioxetine), the authors remarked that new antidepressants have mechanisms of action similar to first- and second-generation antidepressants and there is always a lag phase between the introduction of a drug in the market and the description of withdrawal syndromes.

Box 2.1 New Withdrawal Symptoms After a Decrease or Discontinuation of a SSRI or SNRI

GENERAL: sweating; flu-like symptoms; headache; flushing; chills; fatigue; weakness; pain; malaise; tiredness; lethargy

CARDIOVASCULAR: tachycardia; dizziness; lightheadedness; chest pain; hypertension; postural hypotension; vertigo; syncope; dyspnea

GASTROINTESTINAL: nausea; vomiting; anorexia, appetite problems; diarrhea; abdominal pain/cramp/distention; loose stools; esophagitis; increased bowel movements

SENSORY: electric shock sensations; tinnitus; blurred vision/visual changes; brain zaps; hyperesthesia; altered taste; pruritus; pricking sensations; buzzing noise within the head

NEUROMUSCULAR: paresthesia; myoclonus; tremor; coordination problems; numbness; stiffness; myalgia; ataxia; muscular spasm; neuralgias; jerkiness; arthralgias; cramp; hemiplegia

SEXUAL: premature ejaculation; genital hypersensitivity

NEUROLOGICAL: seizures; stroke-like symptoms

COGNITIVE: confusion; amnesia; decreased concentration; disorientation; lethargy, drowsiness; attention difficulties; slurred speech

AFFECTIVE: anxiety; agitation; depression; irritability; panic; derealization; depersonalization; dysphoria; mood swings; suicidal ideation; hypomania, euphoria; fear; nervousness; tension

BEHAVIORAL: restlessness; aggressive behavior; impulsivity; bouts of crying/outbursts of anger

SLEEP: insomnia; nightmares; sleep problems; vivid dreams; hypersomnia

PSYCHOTIC: visual/auditory hallucinations; delirium; catatonia

---

2. Ketamine and esketamine, that have been approved by the Food and Drug Administration (FDA) for treatment-resistant depression, may be classified at high risk for dependence, addiction, and withdrawal syndromes. The latter typically appear within 24 hours

of discontinuation and are characterized by symptoms such as craving and dysphoria. Cosci and Chouinard (11) challenged their inclusion as antidepressants and I agree with them: in this book, the term "antidepressant medication" does not include ketamine and esketamine.

3. Withdrawal reactions related to discontinuation of antidepressants did not appear to be qualitatively different from those taking place with other psychotropic drugs, such as BZs, antipsychotics, and mood stabilizers. However, only SSRIs, SNRIs, and antipsychotics were consistently associated with persistent postwithdrawal disorders and potentially high severity of syndromes, including alterations of clinical course, whereas the distress associated with BZ discontinuation appeared to be predominantly short-lived.

This latter conclusion, that supports a previous specific review (12), deserves a brief comment. BZs, because of their widespread use and their limited cost, were a major obstacle to the marketing of SSRIs and SNRIs in anxiety disorders. When directly compared to antidepressants in controlled trials, BZs were found to be more or as effective and with fewer side effects (13). In anxious and/or minor depression, BZs were a valid therapeutic option (14). A commercial war was thus started: the dependence potential of BZs was dramatized and their prescription was hindered in all possible ways, despite the clinical value of this class of medication (15). Physicians thus learned that BZs were bad and could cause dependence, whereas antidepressant medications were devoid of such effects. This was probably the most spectacular achievement of propaganda in psychiatry.

Additional insights came from another systematic review on the effects of discontinuation of antidepressants that was published in 2019 (16). The inclusion criteria were articles providing clear, comparable data about the incidence, severity, and duration of withdrawal from antidepressant medications. Unlike previous systematic reviews (8, 9), Davies and Read also included online surveys. This entailed problems in the quality of data collection, but opened the review to a world that was, until then, largely unexplored. The incidence of withdrawal symptoms had wide variations (from 27% to 86%, with a weighted average of 56%). Guidelines on antidepressant use in the UK and USA were not found to incorporate adequate information. Davies and Read (16) also recommended that prescribers should fully inform patients about the possibility of withdrawal effects.

The Definition of Clinical Phenomena Following Discontinuation of Antidepresssant Medications

Upon tapering and discontinuing antidepressant medications, a patient may experience mild distress and symptoms or a disabling withdrawal syndrome. Diagnostic criteria in psychiatry set a threshold for the clinical manifestations of distress, such as anxiety or depression. Criteria for defining withdrawal syndromes from antidepressants were suggested by Black et al., as early as in 2000 (17). Such criteria encompassed both somatic (dizziness, light-headedness, vertigo, shock-like sensations, paresthesias, fatigue, headache, nausea, tremor, diarrhea, visual disturbances) and psychological (anxiety, insomnia, irritability) symptoms and required significant distress to be associated (17). However, only in 2015 was a clear differentiation between withdrawal and other clinical phenomena, such as relapse and rebound, performed (18). Guy and Virginie-Ann Chouinard differentiated the following clinical phenomena:

1. Occurrence of new symptoms that pertain to the list shown in Box 2.1 and may last up to 6 weeks (new withdrawal symptoms).
2. Return of the original symptoms (e.g., anxiety, panic, depression, obsessions) at a greater intensity than before treatment (rebound symptoms).
3. Protraction of new withdrawal symptoms beyond 6 weeks and/or appearance of new symptoms or disorders (persistent postwithdrawal disorder).
4. Reappearance of the episode that was treated with antidepressants (relapse/recurrence).

They formulated diagnostic criteria for the first three clinical manifestations.

Fiammetta Cosci developed a semi-structured research interview for facilitating such assessment that achieved excellent inter-rater agreement (19). Following extensive use of this interview in clinical practice, Cosci and Chouinard (11) subsequently refined the original criteria (18). I am going to describe and discuss the diagnostic criteria for new withdrawal symptoms and persistent postwithdrawal disorder. Since rebound symptoms were found to be of limited importance in our reviews (8, 9) and clinical practice with antidepressant medications (but they appear to be more important with other medications, such as BZs), we refer to the original source (11) for their discussion.

New withdrawal symptoms are usually short-lasting (up to 6 weeks), transient, and reversible. The diagnostic criteria for a withdrawal syndrome (Box 2.2) require the presence of at least two symptoms, but generally a lot more are present. They may occur with any type of antidepressant medication, but particularly with SSRIs and SNRIs. Within SSRIs, paroxetine is the most likely to be associated with withdrawal syndrome, while

---

Box 2.2 Diagnostic Criteria for Withdrawal Syndrome from Antidepressant Medications*

The presence of the following features—that occur with dose decrease, discontinuation, or switch of an antidepressant drug—is required:

1. At least two new withdrawal symptoms (see Box 2.1)—that is, symptoms which were not experienced before starting or during treatment.
2. Symptoms characterized by a peak of onset within 1–10 days after decrease, discontinuation, or switch of an antidepressant medication (depending on drug duration of action) and last for up to 6 weeks (depending on drug elimination half-life).
3. Symptoms cause clinically significant distress.
4. Symptoms are not due to a general medical condition and are not better accounted for by another mental disorder or substance use.

* Modified from references 11 and 18

Source data from Cosci F, Chouinard G: Acute and persistent withdrawal syndromes following discontinuation of psychotropic medications. Psychother Psychosom 2020; 89:283–306.

Chouinard G, Chouinard VA: New classification of selective serotonin reuptake inhibitor withdrawal. Psychother Psychosom 2015; 84:63–71.

fluoxetine appears to be the least likely (8, 11). Within SNRIs, venlafaxine is the most likely to induce withdrawal syndromes (9, 11). Peak of onset may be variable and is influenced by medication half-life: it may occur 36 hours to 7–10 days after drug tapering or discontinuation. I have seen also a few cases in whom new withdrawal symptoms with characteristic manifestations, such as brain zaps, ensued a few months after discontinuation, apparently out of the blue.

Persistent postwithdrawal disorders (Box 2.3) have been described with use of SSRIs and SNRIs medications, as well as with other antidepressants (2–5, 8, 9, 18, 20, 21). Paroxetine and venlafaxine were mostly involved. Their clinical presentation was very variable. At times, such disturbances represent simply the protraction of withdrawal syndromes that occurred upon antidepressant discontinuation. Other times, however, psychiatric symptoms or even disorders emerge that had never occurred before treatment (e.g., a major depressive disorder or cyclothymia

---

Box 2.3 Diagnostic Criteria for Persistent Postwithdrawal Disorder After Antidepressant Discontinuation*

The presence of the following features—that occur with discontinuation or switch of an antidepressant drug—is required:

1. At least two new withdrawal symptoms (see Box 2.1) that were not experienced before the beginning of or during treatment, whose duration exceeds 6 weeks; and/or return of the original symptoms at a greater intensity; and/or appearance of new symptoms/disorders that were not present before.
2. Symptoms cause clinically significant distress.
3. Symptoms are not due to a general medical condition and are not better accounted for by another mental disorder or substance use.

---

* Modified from references 11 and 18.

Source data from Cosci F, Chouinard G: Acute and persistent withdrawal syndromes following discontinuation of psychotropic medications. Psychother Psychosom 2020; 89:283–306.

Chouinard G, Chouinard VA: New classification of selective serotonin reuptake inhibitor withdrawal. Psychother Psychosom 2015; 84:63–71.

in a patient who was treated with antidepressants because of an anxiety disorder and had never experienced mood disturbances before; pathological gambling and generalized anxiety disorder in patients treated for mood disorders without any history of such disturbances) (5, 11, 20). It should be noted that protraction of new withdrawal symptoms shortly after discontinuation of antidepressants does not always characterize postwithdrawal symptomatology: new disorders/disturbances may occur months later without prodromal withdrawal symptomatology. I have also observed that persistent postwithdrawal disorders may have an intermittent course (waves): they fade and apparently disappear, to come back a few months later. These manifestations indicate the complexity and variability of postwithdrawal symptomatology.

The concept of persistent postwithdrawal disorder may also extend to the presence of sexual dysfunction after SSRIs and SNRIs discontinuation (22), that was first described in 2006 (23) and is often referred to as a syndrome called post-SSRI sexual dysfunction (PSSD). The syndrome is characterized by a decrease or absence of libido, genital anesthesia, numbness in nipples, orgasmic disorders (i.e., anorgasmia or anhedonic orgasm), erectile dysfunction, delayed or premature ejaculation, testicular pain or atrophy (in males), lack of lubrication (in females), and by psychological symptoms such as anhedonia, difficulty in concentrating, memory problems, inability to experience sexual attraction to the sight, touch, or idea of a sexual partner (22-25).

The Qualitative Experience of Withdrawal

A couple of years ago, I was lecturing on the sequential model of treatment in an American medical school. During my talk, I mentioned withdrawal reactions from discontinuing antidepressant medications. At the end of the lecture, a medical student of the local university came to me. The situation was very unfavorable for disclosure, but he could not resist from sharing his story. During his pre-med years, he went through a tough time because of the clustering of family, financial, and emotional problems. His primary care physician prescribed sertraline to him. He seemed to get better, passed some exams, and chose to maintain medication for a while. After a couple of years, he decided to stop taking it (he had got into the medical school and things seemed to be looking up), tapering the medication. However, a few days after being drug-free, he went through what he defined as a "dreadful experience." It was not simply having symptoms—he explained to me—it was "unbearable pain." I understood what he meant—mental pain, one of the worst manifestations of suffering (26). He decided not to attempt discontinuation anymore, because he did not want to re-experience those feelings. I only had the time to give him my card and ask him to write to me. He never did. I should have told him that there is a way out; there is a way of decreasing the intensity of symptoms. My missed message was one of the reasons that prompted me to write this book.

References

1. Medawar C: The antidepressant web. Int J Risk Safety Med 1997; 10:75–126.
2. Shoenberger D: Discontinuing paroxetine: a personal account. Psychother Psychosom 2002; 71:237–8.
3. Belaise C, Gatti A, Chouinard VA, Chouinard G: Patient online report of selective serotonin reuptake inhibitor (SSRI) induced persistent postwithdrawal anxiety and mood disorders. Psychother Psychosom 2012; 81:386–8.
4. Bhanji N, Chouinard G, Kolivakis T, Margolese H: Persistent tardive rebound panic disorder, rebound anxiety and insomnia following paroxetine withdrawal: a review of rebound withdrawal phenomena. Can J Clin Pharmacol 2006; 13:69–74.
5. Fava GA, Bernardi M, Tomba E, Rafanelli C: Effects of gradual discontinuation of selective serotonin reuptake inhibitors in panic disorder with agoraphobia. Int J Neuropsychopharmacol 2007; 10:835–8.
6. Guy A, Brown M, Lewis S, Horowitz M: The "patient voice": patients who experience antidepressant withdrawal symptoms are often dismissed, or misdiagnosed with relapse, or a new medical condition. Ther Adv Psychopharmacology 2020 Nov 9; 10:2045125320967183.
7. Fava GA: The decline of pluralism in medicine: dissent is welcome. Psychother Psychosom 2020; 89:1–5.
8. Fava GA, Gatti A, Belaise C, Guidi J, Offidani E: Withdrawal symptoms after selective serotonin reuptake inhibitor discontinuation: a systematic review. Psychother Psychosom 2015; 84:72–81.
9. Fava GA, Benasi G, Lucente M, Offidani E, Cosci F, Guidi J: Withdrawal symptoms after serotonin-noradrenaline reuptake inhibitor discontinuation. Psychother Psychosom 2018; 87:195–203.
10. Hengartner MP, Davies J, Read J: Antidepressant withdrawal—the tide is finally turning. Epidemiol Psych Sci 2019; 29:e52.
11. Cosci F, Chouinard G: Acute and persistent withdrawal syndromes following discontinuation of psychotropic medications. Psychother Psychosom 2020; 89:283–306.

12. Nielsen M, Hansen EH, Goztsche PC: What is the difference between dependence and withdrawal reactions? A comparison of benzodiazepines and selective serotonin re-uptake inhibitors. Addiction 2012; 107:900–8.

13. Offidani E, Guidi J, Tomba E, Fava GA: Efficacy and tolerability of benzodiazepines versus antidepressants in anxiety disorders. Psychother Psychosom 2013; 82:355–62.

14. Benasi G, Guidi J, Offidani E, Balon R, Rickels K, Fava GA: Benzodiazepines as a monotherapy in depressive disorders: a systematic review. Psychother Psychosom 2018; 87:65–74.

15. Balon R, Chouinard G, Cosci F, Dubovsky SL, Fava GA, Freire RC, Greenblatt DJ, Krystal JH, Nardi AE, Rickels K, Roth T, Salzman C, Shader R, Silberman EK, Sonino N, Starcevic V, Weintraub SJ: International Task Force on Benzodiazepines. Psychother Psychosom 2018; 87:193–4.

16. Davies J, Read J: A systematic review into the incidence, severity, and duration of antidepressant withdrawal effects: are guidelines evidence-based? Addictive Behav 2019; 97:111–21.

17. Black K, Shea C, Dursun S, Kutcher S: Selective serotonin reuptake inhibitor discontinuation syndrome: proposed diagnostic criteria. J Psychiatr Neurosci 2000; 25:255–61.

18. Chouinard G, Chouinard VA: New classification of selective serotonin reuptake inhibitor withdrawal. Psychother Psychosom 2015; 84:63–71.

19. Cosci F, Chouinard G, Chouinard V-A, Fava GA: The Diagnostic Clinical Interview for Drug Withdrawal 1(DID-W1)—new symptoms of selective serotonin reuptake inhibitors (SSRI) or serotonin noradrenaline reuptake inhibitors (SNRI): inter-rater reliability. Riv Psichiat 2018; 53:95–9.

20. Belaise C, Gatti A, Chouinard VA, Chouinard G: Persistent postwithdrawal disorders induced by paroxetine, a selective serotonin reuptake inhibitor, and treated with specific cognitive behavioral therapy. Psychother Psychosom 2014; 83:247–8.

21. Stockmann T, Odegbaro D, Timini S, Moncrieff J: SSRI and SNRI withdrawal symptoms reported on an internet forum. Int J Risk Saf Med 2018; 29:175–80.

22. Patacchini A, Cosci F: A paradigmatic case of post-selective serotonin reuptake inhibitors sexual dysfunction or withdrawal after discontinuation of selective serotonin reuptake inhibitors? J Clin Psychopharmacol 2020; 40:93–5.

23. Csoka AB, Shipko S: Persistent sexual side effects after SSRI discontinuation. Psychother Psychosom 2006; 75:187–8.

24. Healy D, Le Noury J, Mangin D: Enduring sexual dysfunctions after treatment with antidepressants, 5-alpha reductase inhibitors and isotretinoin: 300 cases. Int J Risk Saf Med 2018; 29:125–34.

25. Rothmore J: Antidepressant-induced sexual dysfunction. Med J Australia 2020; 212:329–34.

26. Sensky T: Mental pain and suffering. Psychother Psychosom 2020; 89:337–44.

3

The Associated Clinical Manifestations of Behavioral Toxicity

In most instances of diagnostic reasoning in psychiatry, the process ends with the identification of a disorder, often subsumed under a rubric of the *Diagnostic and Statistical Manual of Mental Disorders* (DSM) (1). The diagnostic process could therefore simply lead to a DSM-5 diagnosis of antidepressant discontinuation syndrome, no matter how outdated and imprecise this description, published in 2013. Or it could be expressed in the diagnostic configurations that we described in the previous chapter. However, Alvan Feinstein (2), the father of clinical epidemiology and one of the most important physicians in the USA in the past century, remarks that in medicine, when making a diagnosis, thoughtful clinicians seldom leap from a clinical manifestation to a diagnostic endpoint. Clinical reasoning goes through a series of "transfer stations," where potential connections between presenting symptoms and other clinical manifestations are drawn. These stations are a pause for verification, or a change to another direction (2). As a former student of George Engel, I was taught that clinical observation is the neglected basic method of medicine (3). When dealing with withdrawal reactions from discontinuing antidepressant medications, I was struck by a number of associated clinical features, either at the time of the clinical event or in the patient's history. In analyzing the literature concerned with discontinuing antidepressant medications, I specifically looked for these clinical manifestations.

Associated Clinical Manifestations
of Withdrawal Reactions

In the literature (4–6), a number of clinical phenomena have been found to be associated with withdrawal reactions upon tapering or discontinuation of antidepressant medications: loss of antidepressant efficacy, paradoxical effects, switching to bipolar course, resistance, and refractoriness. Discussion of each clinical event will be preceded by a case illustration from our Affective Disorders Program. Of course, due to a lack of specific studies, we should not forget that the associations could be only casual.

Loss of Clinical Efficacy During Maintenance Treatment

Sarah is a 34-year-old secretary, married with one child. She suffered from recurrent major depressive episodes that responded to antidepressant medication. After the third episode, her primary care physician suggested she continue citalopram 20 mg/day indefinitely. She did well for a couple of years, but then she started having depressive symptoms. Her physician increased citalopram to 40 mg/day, which initially produced some improvement, but then yielded no relief. Sarah was very compliant about her medication and there were no major life events occurring at that time. Her primary care physician referred the patient to our Affective Disorders Program for assessment and treatment. After evaluation, I decided to taper and discontinue citalopram, while Sarah started a sequential combination of cognitive behavior therapy (CBT) and Well-Being Therapy (WBT) (7, 8). During tapering, she experienced withdrawal symptoms (particularly flushing, malaise, brain zaps, and muscular spasms) which reached the threshold of a severe withdrawal syndrome (9) at discontinuation. The syndrome lasted about a month before fading.

The return of depressive symptoms during maintenance antidepressant treatment is a common and vexing clinical problem (10). A patient who is doing well on maintenance pharmacotherapy may have a relapse, despite his/her compliance with medication. In psychiatry, the term "tachyphylaxis" (the progressive reduction in response to a given dose of medication after repeated administration of a pharmacologically or physiologically active substance) has also been used to characterize relapse during maintenance treatment or clinical deterioration marked by symptoms such as apathy and fatigue (11). The use of this term is however questionable, since its Greek root connotes a fast, rapid loss of effect; on the contrary, the phenomenon increases with duration of treatment. In a meta-analysis of maintenance treatment studies, the risk of relapse progressively increased from 23% within 1 year to 34% in 2 years and 45% in 3 years (12). The term "tolerance" would be the most appropriate, but it is carefully avoided because of its potential hints of dependence.

A clinically intuitive strategy for addressing the problem is to increase the dosage of the antidepressant drug, but this therapeutic choice is likely to offer only a temporary solution (13), as was found to be the case with Sarah. However, in two pilot controlled investigations (14, 15), psychotherapy (in one case, the sequential combination of CBT and WBT, and in another, a family intervention), without changing the drug regimen, was significantly more effective than a dose increase in yielding a persistent remission in depressed patients who experienced a loss of clinical effect while being treated with antidepressants. Indeed, Sarah, despite the stormy beginning (her withdrawal syndrome), did well on psychotherapy and achieved enduring remission.

Paradoxical Effects

Emma is a 23-year-old single student of engineering. She became anxious and demoralized about her course of study and future. Her primary care physician prescribed venlafaxine 75 mg/day. In a few weeks she got better. After a few months, however, she developed a deep state of apathy, associated with loss of interest and difficulties falling asleep. Her doctor increased venlafaxine to 150 mg/day. She actually got worse and was referred to our Program. I attributed her apathy to a side effect of venlafaxine (16) and thus decided to taper it with the smallest decrements possible (37.5 mg/day) every other week, while prescribing clonazepam (0.5 mg twice a day). Emma also started the sequential combination of CBT and WBT (7, 8). Upon discontinuation, she went through a severe withdrawal syndrome (characterized by brain zaps, flu-like symptoms, dizziness, hypersensitivity to touch), that developed into a persistent postwithdrawal disorder (9) lasting 3 years. Apathy, however, slowly improved and subsided.

The case illustrates the occurrence of paradoxical effects (such as apathy) during antidepressant treatment, as reported in double-blind placebo-controlled investigations that were concerned with fluoxetine (17) and sertraline (18). Indeed, the concept of antidepressant-induced tardive dysphoria points to the fact that the symptomatology may be reversed by tapering or discontinuing the antidepressant drug (19). In the case of Emma, apathy faded when venlafaxine was stopped, but this does not necessarily occur in every case: paradoxical effects may persist and contribute to a persistent postwithdrawal disorder. Her withdrawal symptoms, however, developed into this syndrome.

During treatment of panic disorder by fluvoxamine (20), the onset of depressive symptoms in 7 of 80 patients (9%) was reported. It is of considerable interest that these patients had no past or current history of depression before fluvoxamine therapy. The symptoms improved when fluvoxamine was stopped and a TCA or clonazepam was substituted as treatment. Depressive symptoms occurred again when fluoxetine was administered (20). Similar observations were made with the use of TCAs in anxiety disorders (21).

In 1968, Alberto Di Mascio et al. (22) investigated the effects of imipramine on individuals who were very heterogeneous as to depression levels, using a double-blind placebo-controlled procedure. Imipramine induced an increase in depression in those with the lowest scores of depression. This landmark early pilot trial suggested the possibility that, when depressive symptoms are minimal, antidepressant medications may do more harm than good.

Switching to Bipolar Course

Robert is a 28-year-old accountant with no past or family history of bipolar disorder, but a characterological tendency to perfectionism and compulsive checking. He is married with no children. Because of some unexpected work changes, these traits progressed into a clearcut obsessive-compulsive disorder, which considerably affected his functioning. His primary care physician prescribed citalopram 20 mg/day, with good results for a few months. Robert, following some positive changes at work, decided to stop taking the antidepressant without consulting his doctor. He first decreased citalopram to 10 mg /day and after two weeks he stopped it. A few days after discontinuation, he presented with both hypomanic symptoms (restlessness, activation, poor sleep, inability to concentrate) and withdrawal manifestations (nausea, diarrhea, stomach cramps, dizziness, palpitations). The symptomatology extended over several weeks, before he decided to look for help.

Treatment with antidepressant medications has been associated with mania or other forms of excessive behavioral activation (23). A systematic review and meta-analysis explored hypomania, mania, and behavioral activation of children and adolescents during antidepressant treatment (24). It disclosed that rates of excessive arousal activation with antidepressants were significantly higher both in anxiety (13.8%) and depression (9.8%), than with placebos (5.2% vs. 1.1%, respectively) (24). As a result, behavioral activation, hypomania, and mania are a consistent risk regardless of individual or family history of bipolar illness. Such risk runs counter to the widespread clinical use of antidepressants in anxiety disorders, particularly in younger patients.

Discontinuation of antidepressant medications may also trigger hypomania or mania, despite concurrent mood-stabilizing treatment (25, 26). The syndrome may be self-limiting, may abate with reinstitution of antidepressant drugs, or may require specific antimanic treatment. Mood elevation may also occur with antidepressant dose decrease (27). In the case of Robert, the syndrome persisted, did not stop with reinstitution of the antidepressant, and required the use of lithium carbonate.

Resistance

Mary is a 56-year-old woman who works in a fashion store. She is married with three children. She suffered from an episode of major depression, a few months after the death of her mother. She was treated with fluoxetine 20 mg/day for 6 months with satisfactory results. Medication was stopped abruptly but no problems ensued. After a year, she started having the same symptoms of the previous episode. Her doctor prescribed fluoxetine again. This time, however, Mary did not respond to the treatment, despite an increase to 40 mg/day. Her doctor decided to change medication and taper fluoxetine, but when it was discontinued (before she had started the new one) she developed a withdrawal syndrome characterized by sweating, palpitations, dizziness, and flu-like symptoms.

The case illustrates the onset of resistance after antidepressant treatment. The term "resistance" is here applied to a lack of response to a previously effective pharmacological treatment when the same medication is started again after a drug-free period (28). It is different from its use for indicating an episode which does not respond to drugs or psychotherapy and is therefore defined as treatment-resistant (29). This latter occurrence, which I am going to discuss under the heading of "refractoriness," is the most common, but also the former takes place in a considerable number of cases (28, 29). In a recent systematic review on the lack of response to rechallenge (28), the range of response failures was broad (between 4.9% and 42.9% across studies). In a large observational study (30), failure to respond to the same medication that was used in a previous episode was found to occur in a quarter of cases. Resistance was examined in a clinical trial of patients who, after initially responding to fluoxetine, were assigned to placebo (31). About half of patients relapsed. After reinitiation of fluoxetine, 38% of depressed patients did not respond at all or displayed an initial response followed by relapse (31).

The data available thus indicate that when drug treatment is reinstituted, the patient may not respond to the same antidepressant which improved depressive symptoms initially. In the case of Mary, it is of considerable interest that she did not develop withdrawal symptoms when fluoxetine was stopped abruptly, but she displayed symptoms of withdrawal, despite tapering, after she had failed to respond to the second trial of fluoxetine. This would seem to indicate not only that resistance and withdrawal are linked, but that the onset of resistance with the second course of fluoxetine heralds a general change in reacting to the antidepressant.

Refractoriness

William is a 48-year-old blue-collar factory worker. He is married with two children. He had a long-standing history of generalized anxiety disorder with an episode of major depressive disorder of recent onset. His primary care physician prescribed paroxetine 20 mg/day. He showed very little response; his doctor increased paroxetine to 40 mg/day. He then switched it to venlafaxine, first at 75 mg/day, then at 150 mg/day, with very little response as to depressive mood and onset of panic attacks. In between the two medications, William had a severe withdrawal reaction.

The ill-defined concept of "treatment resistance" is based on the untested assumption that treatment was right in the first place, and failure to respond is shifted upon patients' characteristics. "Treatment resistance" thus calls for switching and augmentation, as William's physician did. Chiara Rafanelli and I (32) have applied the concept of cascade iatrogenesis—that originated in geriatrics (33)—to psychiatric settings. The patient is prescribed an increasing number of medications that, in the long run, cause other problems and make the illness refractory, instead of reconsidering the treatment selection process.

The Sequenced Treatment Alternatives to Relieve Depression (STAR*D) Study (34) provided an important illustration of this process. The original aim of the trial was to test the best pharmacological strategies for obtaining remission in major depression. Patients entered a first open trial of medication (citalopram), with aggressive dosing and an extended duration of treatment. Only 37% of patients reached remission (34). Patients who did not recover after the first trial of medication were submitted to three sequential steps involving switching, augmentation, or combination strategies, based on existing evidence. The cumulative rate of remission, after all four sequential steps, was 67%; however, when persistent recovery (also including relapse rates while on treatment) was considered, the cumulative rate was 43%. Therapeutic efforts after step one (open treatment with citalopram) yielded only an additional 6% of sustained recovery. Remission rates decreased after each treatment step, despite the fact that each step of the trial was carefully conceived to increase the likelihood of response in patients who did not remit (34). In each sequential treatment step, the rates of relapse (while still on medication) increased in patients who achieved remission. Further, after each treatment step, intolerance to treatment increased (as evidenced by dropouts for any reason during the first 4 weeks, or side effects afterwards).

Prior use of antidepressant medications, but not of psychotherapy (35), has been found to be related to both resistance and refractoriness (35–37).

Behavioral Toxicity and Iatrogenic Comorbidity

Withdrawal syndromes and persistent postwithdrawal disorders may thus be associated with loss of antidepressant efficacy, paradoxical effects, switching to bipolar course, resistance, and refractoriness (5, 6, 9). But all these manifestations may also be related to each other. Raja (38) described nine patients who had an initial good response to treatment with antidepressant drugs. However, such response was followed by loss of efficacy, resistance, and worsening with subsequent treatment. These manifestations appeared to be closely connected and part of the same syndrome. Sharma (39) described how patients who displayed loss of efficacy during maintenance treatment with antidepressants subsequently developed refractoriness. In patients who respond to the same medication that was used in the previous episode, a loss of therapeutic effect may then ensue (30). Bader and Dunner (40) pointed to the association between antidepressant-induced mania and treatment-refractory depression in patients who lacked a family history of bipolar disorder. All these interrelationships suggest that withdrawal reactions may be connected with other clinical manifestations, be part of the same syndrome, and have a common underlying mechanism.

In 1968, Alberto Di Mascio and associates introduced the concept of behavioral toxicity of psychotropic drugs (41–43). It referred to the pharmacological actions of a drug that, within the dose range in which it has been found to possess clinical utility, may produce alterations in mood and in perceptual, cognitive, and psychomotor functions that limit the capacity of the individual or constitute a hazard to his/her well-being. The use of the term "toxicity" was not conventional, since it was not restricted to immediately dangerous clinical effects such as in overdose or to drugs with narrow therapeutic indices, such as lithium. Di Mascio et al. (42) described two major drug-induced mood changes. "Paradoxical" drug effects are those alterations in mood in a direction opposite to the clinically desirable, such as increased anxiety and rage with BZs and deepening of depression with antidepressant drugs (42, 43). "Pendular" drug effects are those alterations that proceed in a desired direction, however to a degree that the resultant state tends toward the opposite condition for which the drug was initially administered, such as euphoria with antidepressant drugs (42, 43). These important conceptual papers (41–43) were published in a journal, *Connecticut Medicine*, that did not have sufficient visibility. Not surprisingly, their formulation received scant attention in the literature, until our research group drew attention to it in 2016 (44).

Indeed, the concept of behavioral toxicity may provide a unifying framework for all the manifestations we described before, and explain their interrelationships and variability. Behavioral toxicity may play a key role in the process of balancing the benefits of a potential treatment, by consideration of the potential adverse events that may be triggered by the therapeutic act. Indeed, Di Mascio and Shader (41) noted that a drug effect, such as sedation or motor stimulation, may be considered adverse for one patient, and yet therapeutic and desired for another patient; within the same patient, it may be of value at one stage of his/her illness, but adverse at a later stage.

The concept of behavioral toxicity may demarcate major prognostic and therapeutic differences. Medications of the same class may be equally effective, but may entail different risks of behavioral toxicity. For instance, paroxetine and venlafaxine appear to be associated with higher risks of dependence and onset of withdrawal reactions compared to other SSRIs (5) or SNRIs (6). Dual reuptake inhibitors (TCAs and venlafaxine) were found to yield lower rates of loss of efficacy than SSRIs (45). Another example may be provided when withdrawal symptoms are misunderstood as indicators of impending relapse and lead to unnecessary reinstitution of treatment (44). They may worsen the state of behavioral toxicity, with subsequent episodes of refractoriness to treatment. Refractoriness to treatment, in turn, lends itself to the use of switching and/or augmenting strategies which, as STAR*D teaches (34), may propel depressive illness into a phase characterized by low remission, high relapse, and high intolerance to medications.

The concept of behavioral toxicity, however, does not provide differentiation between adverse events that are limited to the period of psychotropic drug administration and effects that may persist long after their discontinuation. These latter phenomena led to the introduction of the concept of iatrogenic comorbidity (44), that refers to the unfavorable modifications in the course, characteristics, and responsiveness to treatment of an illness that may be related to previously administered therapies (29, 32, 44). Such vulnerabilities may manifest themselves during treatment administration and/or after its discontinuation. The changes are persistent and not limited to a short phase such as in most of the cases of withdrawal syndromes.

Iatrogenic Comorbidity in Childhood and Adolescence

All manifestations of behavioral toxicity secondary to antidepressant medications (including withdrawal reactions) may occur in childhood and adolescence (46). Indeed, for some of them (switching to bipolar course) there is evidence suggesting that they may be more severe and frequent than in adulthood (24). We reported the following case (46), which may be indicative of the seriousness of the phenomena.

Ann is a 14-year-old girl who developed school phobia at the beginning of high school. Her parents brought her to a child psychiatrist who prescribed citalopram (20 mg/day). After one month, she was still refusing to go back to school and the psychiatrist added alprazolam (0.25 mg twice a day). As one would have expected from the available literature, there was no response to this drug combination. Ann's parents thus decided to consult with me. I immediately referred her for CBT with an experienced psychologist. Since it was spring, and I feared withdrawal problems with both drugs, I did not stop the two medications, postponing drug tapering and discontinuation to the end of the school year (June). After the first session of psychotherapy, Ann was back to school, and with weekly sessions over a period of 3 months she was able to complete the school year. I then tapered and discontinued alprazolam first, and citalopram later. In both cases, withdrawal symptoms emerged, but they were far more severe and persisting after citalopram discontinuation (nervousness, agitation, sleep problems, and suicidal ideation for about 6 weeks), despite the ongoing psychotherapy. Ann successfully completed high school and did not present problems at a 4-year follow-up.

The case illustrates the severity of withdrawal syndromes that may ensue after only a few months of treatment with citalopram. It also cautions about the use of antidepressant medications in childhood and adolescence (46).

The Spectrum of Comorbidity

Alvan Feinstein's definition of comorbidity as "any distinct additional clinical entity that has existed or that may occur during the clinical course of a patient who has the index disease under study" referred also to antecedent pathological events that were judged to affect the current disease process (47). The cross-sectional nature of the classification systems in psychiatry has limited the use of the term "comorbidity" to what a patient may be currently experiencing and to co-occurring diagnostic entities, and yet the role of iatrogenic comorbidity is clear in everyday practice. For instance, when antidepressant drugs trigger a manic or hypomanic episode in allegedly unipolar disorders (i.e., patients who do not have a family or personal history of bipolar illness or similar manifestations), discontinuation of the medication is unlikely to offer a solution to the problem, which tends to persist and modify the entire course of illness in a cascade of affective episodes (44).

The concepts of behavioral toxicity and iatrogenic comorbidity provide very helpful descriptions of clinical phenomena, but not an explanation as to why they occur. As the pharmacologist David Grahame-Smith once remarked: "Chronic drug therapy may induce a sleeping tiger, which awakens when the drug therapy is stopped and results in rebound withdrawal effects with serious consequences, as with many drug addictions" (48, p. 227). But what is this "sleeping tiger" in pathophysiological terms?

References

1. Diagnostic and Statistical Manual of Mental Disorders: Fifth Edition. DSM-5. Washington, DC, American Psychiatric Association, 2013.
2. Feinstein AR: An analysis of diagnostic reasoning. I. The domains and disorders of clinical macrobiology. Yale J Biol Med 1973; 46:212–32.
3. Engel GL: Clinical observation: the neglected basic method of medicine. JAMA 1965; 192:849–52.
4. Fava GA: Can long-term treatment with antidepressant drugs worsen the course of depression? J Clin Psychiatry 2003; 64:123–33.
5. Fava GA, Gatti A, Belaise C, Guidi J, Offidani E: Withdrawal symptoms after selective serotonin reuptake inhibitor discontinuation: a systematic review. Psychother Psychosom 2015; 84:72–81.

6. Fava GA, Benasi G, Lucente M, Offidani E, Cosci F, Guidi J: Withdrawal symptoms after serotonin-noradrenaline reuptake inhibitor discontinuation. Psychother Psychosom 2018; 87:195–203.
7. Fava GA: Well-Being Therapy: Treatment Manual and Clinical Applications. Basel, Karger, 2016.
8. Fava GA, Cosci F, Guidi J, Tomba E: Well-being therapy in depression: new insights into the role of psychological well-being in the clinical process. Depr Anxiety 2017; 34:801–8.
9. Cosci F, Chouinard G: Acute and persistent withdrawal syndromes following discontinuation of psychotropic medications. Psychother Psychosom 2020; 89:283–306.
10. Fornaro M, Anastasia A, Novello S, Fusco A, Pariano R, De Berardis D, Solmi M, Veronese N, Stubbs B, Vieta E, Berk M, de Bartolomeis A, Carvalho AF: The emergence of loss of efficacy during antidepressant drug treatment for major depressive disorder. Pharmacol Res 2019; 139:494–503.
11. Kinrys G, Gold AK, Pisano VD, Freeman MP, Papakostas GI, Mischoulon DS, Nierenberg AA, Fava M: Tachyphylaxis in major depressive disorder. J Affect Disord 2019; 245:488–97.
12. Williams N, Simpson AN, Simpson K, Nahas Z. Relapse rates with long-term antidepressant drug therapy: a meta-analysis. Hum Psychopharmacol 2009; 24:401–8.
13. Schmidt ME, Fava M, Zhang S, Gonzales J, Raute NJ, Judge R: Treatment approaches to major depressive disorder relapse. Part I: dose increase. Psychother Psychosom 2002; 71:190–4.
14. Fava GA, Ruini C, Rafanelli C, Grandi S: Cognitive behavior approach to loss of clinical effect during long-term antidepressant treatment: a pilot study. Am J Psychiatry 2002; 159:2094–5.
15. Fabbri S, Fava GA, Rafanelli C, Tomba E: Family intervention approach to loss of clinical effect during long-term antidepressant treatment: a pilot study. J Clin Psychiatry 2007; 68:1348–51.
16. Rothschild AJ: The Rothschild scale for antidepressant tachyphylaxis: reliability and validity. Compr Psychiatry 2008; 49:508–13.
17. Cusin C, Fava M, Amsterdam JD, Quitkin FM, Reimherr FW, Beasley CM, Rosenbaum JF, Perlis RH: Early symptomatic worsening during treatment with fluoxetine in major depressive disorder: prevalence and implications. J Clin Psychiatry 2007; 68:52–7.
18. Harvey AT, Silkey BS, Kornstein SG, Quitkin F: Acute worsening of chronic depression during a double-blind, randomized clinical trial of antidepressant efficacy: differences by sex and menopausal status. J Clin Psychiatry 2007; 68:951–8.
19. El-Mallakh RS, Gao Y, Briscoe BT, Clary CM: Antidepressant induced tardive dysphoria. Psychother Psychosom 2011; 80:57–9.
20. Fux M, Taub M, Zohar J: Emergence of depressive symptoms during treatment for panic disorder with specific 5-hydroxytryptophan reuptake inhibitors. Acta Psychiatr Scand 1993; 88:235–7.
21. Noyes R, Garvey HJ, Cook BL: Follow-up study of patients with panic disorder and agoraphobia with panic attacks treated with tricyclic antidepressants. J Affect Disord 1989; 16:249–57.

22. Di Mascio A, Meyer RE, Stifler L: Effects of imipramine on individuals varying in level of depression. Am J Psychiatry 1968; 127:55-8.
23. Tondo L, Vázquez G, Baldessarini RJ: Mania associated with antidepressant treatment: comprehensive meta-analytic review. Acta Psychiatr Scand 2010; 121:404-14.
24. Offidani E, Fava GA, Tomba E, Baldessarini RJ: Excessive mood elevation and behavioral activation with antidepressant treatment of juvenile depressive and anxiety disorders. Psychother Psychosom 2013; 82:132-41.
25. Landry P, Roy L: Withdrawal hypomania associated with paroxetine. J Clin Psychopharmacol 1997; 17:60-1.
26. Andrade C: Antidepressant-withdrawal mania. J Clin Psychiatry 2004; 65:987-93.
27. Corral M, Sivertz K, Jones BD: Transient mood elevation associated with antidepressant drug decrease. Can J Psychiatry 1987; 32:764-7.
28. Bosman RC, Waumans RC, Jacobs GE, Oude Voshar RC, Muntingh ADT, Van Balkom AJLM: Failure to respond after reinstatement of antidepressant medication: a systematic review. Psychother Psychosom 2018; 87:268-75.
29. Fava GA, Cosci F, Guidi J, Rafanelli C: The deceptive manifestations of treatment resistance in depression. Psychother Psychosom 2020; 89:265-73.
30. Solomon DA, Leon AC, Mueller TI, Coryell W, Teres JL, Posternak MA, Judd LL, Endicott J, Keller MB: Tachyphylaxis in unipolar major depressive disorder. J Clin Psychiatry 2005; 66:283-290.
31. Fava M, Schmidt ME, Zhang S, Gonzales J, Raute NJ, Judge R: Treatment approaches to major depressive disorder relapse. Part II. Re-initiation of antidepressant treatment. Psychother Psychosom 2002; 71:195-9.
32. Fava GA, Rafanelli C: Iatrogenic factors in psychopathology. Psychother Psychosom 2019; 88:129-40.
33. Thornlow DK, Anderson R, Oddone E: Cascade iatrogenesis: factors leading to the development of adverse events in hospitalized older adults. Int J Nurs Stud 2009; 46:1528-35.
34. Rush AJ, Trivedi MH, Wisniewski SR, Nierenberg AA, Stewart JW, Warden D, Niederehe G, Thase ME, Lavori PW, Lebowitz BD, McGrath PJ, Rosenbaum JF, Sackeim HA, Kupfer DJ, Luther J, Fava M: Acute and longer-term outcomes in depressed outpatients requiring one or several treatment steps: a STAR*D report. Am J Psychiatry 2006; 163:1905-17.
35. Leykin Y, Amsterdam JD, DeRubeis RJ, Gallopp R, Shelton RC, Hollon SD: Progressive resistance to a selective serotonin reuptake inhibitor but not to cognitive therapy in the treatment of major depression. J Consult Clin Psychol 2007; 75:267-76.
36. Amsterdam JD, Williams D, Michelson D, Adler LA, Dunner DL, Nierenberg AA, Reimherr FW, Schatzberg AF: Tachyphylaxis after repeated antidepressant drug exposure in patients with recurrent major depressive disorder. Neuropsychobiology 2009; 59:227-33.
37. Amsterdam JD, Kim TT: Prior antidepressant treatment trials may predict a greater risk of depressive relapse during antidepressant maintenance therapy. J Clin Psychopharmacol 2019; 39:344-50.

38. Raja M: Delayed loss of efficacy and depressogenic action of antidepressants. J Clin Psychopharmacol 2009; 29:612–14.
39. Sharma V: Loss of response to antidepressants and subsequent refractoriness. J Affect Disord 2001; 64:99–106.
40. Bader CD, Dunner DL: Antidepressant-induced hypomania in treatment-resistant depression. J Psychiatr Pract 2007; 13:233–7.
41. Di Mascio A, Shader RI: Behavioral toxicity of psychotropic drugs. I. Definition. II. Toxic effect on psychomotor function. Conn Med 1968; 32:617–20.
42. Di Mascio A, Giller DR, Shader RI: Behavioral toxicity of psychotropic drugs. III. Effect on perceptual and cognitive functions. IV. Effect on emotional (mood) states. Conn Med 1968; 32:771–5.
43. Di Mascio A, Shader RI, Harmatz GS: Behavioral toxicity of psychotropic drugs. V. Effects on gross behavioral patterns. Conn Med 1968; 33:279–81.
44. Fava GA, Cosci F, Offidani J, Guidi J: Behavioral toxicity revisited. J Clin Psychopharmacol 2016; 36:550–3.
45. Posternak MA, Zimmerman M: Dual reuptake inhibitors incur lower rates of tachyphylaxis than selective serotonin reuptake inhibitors. J Clin Psychiatry 2005; 66:705–7.
46. Offidani E, Fava GA, Sonino N: Iatrogenic comorbidity in childhood and adolescence. CNS Drugs 2014; 28:769–74.
47. Feinstein AR: The pre-therapeutic classification of comorbidity in chronic disease. J Chronic Dis 1970; 23:455–68.
48. Grahame-Smith DG: "Keep on taking the tablets." Pharmacological adaptation during long-term drug therapy. Br J Clin Pharmacol. 1997; 42:227–38.

4

Understanding the Pathophysiology of Withdrawal Syndromes

The clinical events that may follow tapering and/or discontinuation of antidepressant medications are very variable: they may range from no or limited withdrawal symptoms to severe withdrawal syndromes; they may occur within days, if not hours or have a delayed onset; they may fade away or persist for months or years, accompanied by new disorders and/ or greater intensity of the original disturbance. Further, withdrawal and persistent postwithdrawal disorders may be associated with other manifestations of behavioral toxicity, such as loss of clinical efficacy, paradoxical effects, switching to bipolar course, resistance, and refractoriness. When phenomena are complex and clinical presentations differ so much from each other, the conceptual model used by the clinician affects the interpretation of phenomena and the selection of management strategies to a great extent (1).

In terms of pathophysiology, we may have distinct and yet ostensibly related mechanisms or all these manifestations may be part of the same pathway. If we try to view the clinical phenomena that have been described under a unifying light, we should necessarily refer to the concept of tolerance (2). There are two main forms of tolerance: one is pharmacokinetic (decreased concentrations of the drug in the blood for various metabolic reasons); the other is pharmacodynamic (interaction with receptors) (3). Pharmacokinetics includes processes such as absorption, distribution, blood levels, transformation, and secretion; pharmacodynamics encompasses the physiological effects of a drug, such as therapeutic and adverse effects, as well as the body's compensatory adjustments to the presence of the drug.

Pharmacokinetic models of tolerance have a very limited explanatory power as to the clinical phenomena previously described, even though they can definitely play a role in certain manifestations. Withdrawal syndromes are particularly frequent with short-elimination half-life antidepressant medications, such as paroxetine and venlafaxine, and less frequent with long-elimination half-life medications, such as fluoxetine (4–7). Thus, a pharmacokinetic model may provide the conceptual background for gradual tapering and the switch from short-elimination half-life antidepressants to fluoxetine. Gradual reduction of antidepressant drugs may allow time for the adaptation of the system to lowered levels of the ligand, limiting withdrawal symptomatology (7). The pharmacokinetic model, however, is unable to explain the duration of withdrawal manifestations, with particular reference to persistent postwithdrawal disorders associated with the return of the original illness at a greater intensity than before treatment and/or the occurrence of psychiatric disorders that never occurred before (4, 5, 8). Pharmacokinetic mechanisms cannot be advocated for the appearance and link of other manifestations of behavioral toxicity that are associated with withdrawal and postwithdrawal disturbances, such as the onset of hypomania, loss of clinical effects, and refractoriness to treatment.

I thus thought that pharmacodynamic models that indicate changes in drug-sensitive systems could be more suitable for explaining the manifestations of behavioral toxicity.

The Oppositional Model of Tolerance

Antidepressant drugs are characterized by a delayed onset of therapeutic benefits until 3–4 weeks. It is widely recognized (9, 10) that adaptive responses, such as 5HT2A receptor changes or 5HT4 receptor binding, which are different from the initial ones, mediate therapeutic actions at 3–4 weeks. Such adaptive changes may take place through 5HT1A autoreceptor activity and/or be associated with the allosteric modulation of the serotonin transporter protein that was detected with SSRIs such as paroxetine and escitalopram (11). However, for some strange reason, it is generally assumed that no further adaptive changes may occur after 3–4 weeks and when antidepressant drugs are discontinued everything goes back to the pretreatment state. This is very unlikely, as an analysis of the onset of side effects from antidepressant treatment may teach (12). For instance, SSRIs may induce a decrease of appetite in the first months of treatment, but this effect is substituted by increased appetite and weight gain afterward (12). Similarly, antidepressant medications may have short-term anti-inflammatory effects, but they tend to increase inflammation in the long term (13).

Pharmacodynamic tolerance is a complex and only partially explored phenomenon (14). Two general models have been advanced (15). One model postulates that tolerance results from a reduction in the drug signal or stimulus at the receptor level (e.g., receptor down-regulation or sensitization). The second model postulates that the initial effects of a drug are opposed or counteracted by homeostatic changes in biochemical and cellular systems (e.g., post-receptor signal transduction, neuronal architecture) (15). This latter model was used for the understanding of clinical phenomena related to drugs such as opiates and amphetamines (15) but, after examining it, I thought it was very suitable for understanding the mechanisms and side effects of antidepressant medications (16).

According to the oppositional model of tolerance, continued drug treatment may stimulate processes that run counter to the initial acute effects of a drug (15–17). Such processes may involve the complex balance of serotonin receptors. Adaptive responses, such as 5HT2A receptor changes or 5HT4 receptor binding, which are different from the initial ones, may modulate oppositional effects (17). Various genetic polymorphisms in serotonin receptors (including the 5HT1A, 5HT1B, and 5HT2 subtypes) may have a role in determining the extent to which opposing and compensatory processes occur in response to the initial effects of drugs (18). Environmental factors, such as stressful life circumstances, may also affect this balance and may have an epigenetic role (19). Further, factors such as the duration and type of treatment, prior history of exposure to antidepressant drugs, and pharmacological manipulations such as augmenting and switch strategies may have very profound implications as well (16, 17). The duration of such changes may be variable: if persistent, the changes may cause unfavorable modifications in the trajectory, characteristics, and responsiveness to subsequent treatment of the illness (16, 17).

The oppositional model of tolerance related to antidepressant medications was first presented in 1999 (16) and underwent subsequent updates (17, 20, 21). It may have three different phases of application: early treatment, long-term treatment, and the phase after antidepressant discontinuation (Figure 4.1).

In the early phase of treatment (up to 6 weeks), oppositional processes may cause hypomania/mania or paradoxical reactions such as deepening of depression. With long-term therapy, loss of treatment efficacy and some side effects (such as increased appetite and weight gain), which did not occur initially, may then appear (17). These mechanisms may also lead the illness to a treatment-unresponsive course. When drug treatment ends, oppositional processes no longer meet resistance, resulting in the potential onset of new withdrawal symptoms, persistent postwithdrawal disorders, hypomania, and resistance to treatment if it is reinstituted. In the long run, antidepressant medications may increase chronicity and vulnerability to depressive disorders, constituting a form of iatrogenic comorbidity.

The oppositional model of tolerance is complex and multifactorial and is influenced by the duration of and prior exposure to antidepressant treatment, as well as by psychosocial and genetic factors. As a result, the presence, duration, and characteristics of oppositional processes may vary from one antidepressant to another, from person to person, and even from one episode to another of the use of the same antidepressant

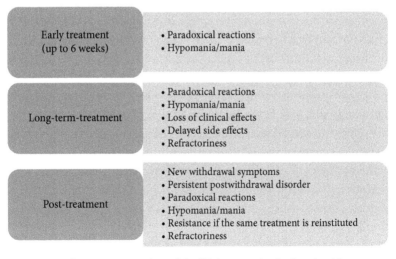

Figure 4.1 The Oppositional Model of Tolerance Applied to Antidepressant Medications

in the same person. The model is realistic instead of idealistic and provides a unifying interpretation of clinical events that otherwise would be scattered and meaningless. Even though it has not been formally tested in experimental studies (including at the preclinical level), it has been supported by a growing number of clinical investigations that have taken place over the past two decades (16, 17, 20, 21). Further, in my clinical practice, I have found that it provides a practical framework for understanding and predicting events that may ensue with antidepressant drugs.

Implications for the Long-Term Outcome of Depression

In addition to the various manifestations of behavioral toxicity that I have discussed in the previous chapter, one of the consequences of the oppositional forces that are triggered by treatment with antidepressant drugs may be a higher likelihood of relapse with prolongation of treatment. Indeed, Viguera and colleagues (22) analyzed 27 studies with variable length of antidepressant treatment and follow-up upon drug discontinuation. When one more study (23) was included, the risk of post-discontinuation relapse was nearly significantly greater after long treatment following recovery from an index episode of major depression (2). Amsterdam and Kim (24) found that the more the number of previous antidepressant trials, the higher the risk of depressive relapse during antidepressant maintenance treatment.

Yet, prolongation of pharmacological treatments to maintain the clinical responses obtained in the short term is advocated for relapse prevention in depression (25), and this conviction is shared by the majority of physicians. The basic assumption is that prolongation of the treatment that yielded remission is the best strategy to prevent relapse of depression. The evidence supporting this strategy, however, is mainly based on clinical trials where remitted patients were randomized to drug continuation or placebo, without any differentiation between withdrawal and relapse. Such an assumption has recently been challenged (26–29): we have no way to know how many of the relapses were actually withdrawal and postwithdrawal syndromes in the group that underwent drug tapering and discontinuation. Further, patients with multiple depressive episodes experience significantly less benefit in relapse prevention during the antidepressant maintenance phase compared to those with a single episode (30). This means that prolongation of antidepressant therapy is unlikely to be effective just when relapse prevention is most needed (recurrent depression).

The length of the first antidepressant treatment was studied in relation to relapse in a sample of 9,243 patients treated with SSRIs (31). Subjects were followed up for 5 years and divided into early discontinuers (who discontinued antidepressant drugs within 6 months), continuing users (who received antidepressants for 6 to 12 months), and persistent users (who were treated with antidepressants for more than 12 months). No differences were found in time to recurrence between patients who were treated for 6 months and those treated for 6 to 12 months. Those who received antidepressant medications for more than a year showed a 23% higher risk of experiencing a second episode than early discontinuers. These results were also confirmed in a subsequent study reporting no differences in risk of relapse between early discontinuers and continuing antidepressant users (32). This means that the longer the duration of antidepressant treatment, the more likely were the episodes to recur. In other longitudinal naturalistic studies involving all types of antidepressants, a higher incidence and longer duration of episodes of major depression was found in those who used antidepressants compared to those not taking those medications (33). Even though the results might have been confounded by the possibility that antidepressants were prescribed to the most severe and recurring cases, the impact of antidepressant medications in the general population did not appear to be favorable (33).

Recovery as a One-Way Street

Antidepressant medications were developed and found to be effective in the treatment of severe depression, but the better tolerability of newer antidepressant drugs has stretched their original indications to milder forms of mood disturbances. Their use has been prolonged to maintenance and prevention of relapse of depression (34). However, if treatment is prolonged beyond 6 months, phenomena such as tolerance, episode acceleration, sensitization, and paradoxical effects may ensue. The hidden costs of using the antidepressant medications may then outweigh their apparent gains, particularly when the likelihood of responsiveness is low (34).

There is clearly the need of a paradigm shift in research on antidepressants. There are major conceptual and clinical issues that may originate from research on behavioral toxicity of antidepressant drugs, including withdrawal syndromes. A hidden conceptual assumption of a large body of research on treatment in depression is that, with appropriate treatment, depressive disturbances will go back to a premorbid state—that is, the receptor changes that are induced by antidepressant medications are limited to their time of administration or shortly afterward, and that it is just a matter of allowing time for adaptation of the system to antidepressant discontinuation. This naïve assumption runs counter to current concepts on the plasticity of the brain (19). The literature that my group and I surveyed and, in particular, the oppositional model of tolerance, suggest that remission and recovery in mood disorders are a one-way street, characterized by structural remodeling of neural architecture and continually changing patterns of gene expression mediated by epigenetic mechanisms (19).

Often patients who undergo painful withdrawal experiences regret and ruminate on the time when an antidepressant was first prescribed. Emma, the engineer student whose case I described in the previous chapter, remarked: "It is clear to me now that I did not need the prescription of venlafaxine. I was simply going through a tough time. That 'original sin' has destroyed my life and affected all my years after. Shall I ever be back to the way I was before?" My answer was: "There is no way back, but there is a way out. And you can become much better than you were before."

References

1. Fava GA, Belaise C: Discontinuing antidepressant drugs. Psychother Psychosom 2018; 87:257–67.
2. Baldessarini RJ, Ghaemi SN, Viguera AC: Tolerance in antidepressant treatment. Psychother Psychosom 2002; 71:177–9.
3. Maxwell SRJ: Pharmacodynamics for the prescriber. Medicine 2016; 44:401–6.

4. Fava GA, Gatti A, Belaise C, Guidi J, Offidani E: Withdrawal symptoms after selective serotonin reuptake inhibitor discontinuation: a systematic review. Psychother Psychosom 2015; 84:72–81.
5. Fava GA, Benasi G, Lucente M, Offidani E, Cosci F, Guidi J: Withdrawal symptoms after serotonin-noradrenaline reuptake inhibitor discontinuation. Psychother Psychosom 2018; 87:195–203.
6. Rosenbaum JF, Fava M, Hoog SL, Ascroft C, Krebs WB: Selective serotonin reuptake inhibitor discontinuation syndrome: a randomized clinical trial. Biol Psychiatry 1998; 44:77–87.
7. Horowitz MA, Taylor D: Tapering of SSRI treatment to mitigate withdrawal symptoms. Lancet Psychiatry 2019; 6:538–46.
8. Cosci F, Chouinard G: Acute and persistent withdrawal syndromes following discontinuation of psychotropic medications. Psychother Psychosom 2020; 89:283–306.
9. Grahame-Smith DG: "Keep on taking the tablets." Pharmacological adaptation during long-term drug therapy. Br J Clin Pharmacol. 1997; 42:227–38.
10. Cosci F, Chouinard G: The monoamine hypothesis of depression revisited: could it mechanistically novel antidepressant strategies? In: Quevedo J, Carvalho AF, Zarate CA (eds). Neurobiology of Depression: Road to Novel Therapeutics. London, UK, Elsevier, 2019, pp. 63–73.
11. Coleman JA, Green EM, Gouax E: X-ray structures and mechanism of the human serotonin transporter. Nature 2016; 532:334–9.
12. Carvalho AF, Sharma MS, Brunoni AR, Vieta E, Fava GA: The safety, tolerability and risks associated with the use of newer generation antidepressant drugs: a critical review of the literature. Psychother Psychosom 2016; 85:270–88.
13. Littrell JL: Taking the perspective that a depressive state reflects inflammation: implications for the use of antidepressants. Front Psychol 2012; 3:297.
14. Bespalov A, Muller R, Relo AL, Hudzik T: Drug tolerance: a known unknown in translational neuroscience. Trend Pharmacol Sci 2016; 37:364–78.
15. Young AM, Goudie AJ: Adaptive processes regulating tolerance to behavioral effects of drugs. In: Bloom FE, Kupfer DJ (eds). Psychopharmacology. New York, Raven Press, 1995, pp. 733–42.
16. Fava GA: Potential sensitizing effects of antidepressant drugs on depression. CNS Drugs 1999; 12:247–56.
17. Fava GA: May antidepressant drugs worsen the conditions they are supposed to treat? The clinical foundations of the oppositional model of tolerance. Ther Adv Psychopharmacol 2020; 10:2045125320970325.
18. Shapiro BB: Subtherapeutic doses of SSRI antidepressants demonstrate considerable serotonin transporter occupancy: implications for tapering SSRIs. Psychopharmacology 2018;235:2779–81.
19. McEwen BS: Epigenetic interactions and the brain-body communication. Psychother Psychosom 2017; 86:1–4.
20. Fava GA: Can long-term treatment with antidepressant drugs worsen the course of depression? J Clin Psychiatry 2003; 64:123–33.
21. Fava GA, Offidani E: The mechanisms of tolerance in antidepressant action. Progr Neuro-Psychopharmacol Biol Psychiatry 2011; 35:1593–602.

22. Viguera AC, Baldessarini RJ, Friedberg J: Discontinuing antidepressant treatment in major depression. Harvard Rev Psychiatry 1998; 5:293–306.
23. Schmidt ME, Fava M, Zhang S, Gonzales J, Raute NJ, Judge R: Treatment approaches to major depressive disorder relapse. Part I: dose increase. Psychother Psychosom 2002; 71:190–4.
24. Amsterdam JD, Kim TT: Prior antidepressant treatment trials may predict a greater risk of depressive relapse during antidepressant maintenance therapy. J Clin Psychopharmacol 2019; 39:344–50.
25. American Psychiatric Association. Practice guideline for the treatment of patients with major depressive disorder. Third edition. Am J Psychiatry 2010; 167 (Suppl):1–118.
26. Baldessarini RJ, Tondo L: Effects of treatment discontinuation in clinical psychopharmacology. Psychother Psychosom 2019; 88:65–70.
27. Cohen D, Recalt AM: Discontinuing psychotropic drugs from participants in randomized controlled trials. Psychother Psychosom 2019; 88:96–104.
28. Recalt AM, Cohen S: Withdrawal confounding in randomized controlled trials of antipsychotic, antidepressant, and stimulant drugs, 2000–2017. Psychother Psychosom 2019; 88:105–13.
29. Hengartner M: How effective are antidepressants for depression over the long-term? Ther Adv Psychopharmacol 2020 May 8; 10:2045125320921694.
30. Kaymaz N, van Os J, Loonen AJ, Nolen WA: Evidence that patients with single versus recurrent depressive episodes are differentially sensitive to treatment discontinuation: a meta-analysis of placebo-controlled randomized trials. J Clin Psychiatry 2008; 69:1423–36.
31. Gardarsdottir H, van Geffen EC, Stolker JJ, Egberts TC, Heerdink ER: Does the length of the first antidepressant treatment episode influence risk and time to a second episode? J Clin Psychopharmacol 2009; 29:69–72.
32. Gardarsdottir H, Egberts TC, Stolker JJ, Heerdink ER: Duration of antidepressant drug treatment and its influence on risk of relapse/recurrence: immortal and neglected time bias. Am J Epidemiol 2009; 170:280–5.
33. Patten SB: The impact of antidepressant treatment on population health. Pop Health Metrics 2004; 2:9.
34. Fava GA: Rational use of antidepressant drugs. Psychother Psychosom 2014; 83:197–204.

5

The Decision
to Discontinue Antidepressants

Discontinuing antidepressant medications is always a complex decision that is frequently much more difficult than their simple prescription. Ideally, it should take place in a setting of shared decision-making between the physician and the patient (1). Such a process involves defining the problem for decision analysis, identifying alternatives, and creating a constructive environment in terms of timing, attention, and communication style (including the language around medications) (1). As Gupta, Miller, and Cahill remark in their book on deprescribing (1), both the physician and the patient are experts, the latter "by experience." However, in practice, these collaborative conditions are seldom met. The physician is often guided by unrealistic attitudes and misleading information skewed by pharmaceutical propaganda and does not have the necessary information for decision analysis.

Despite the fact that self-rating scales are recognized as an important component of psychopharmacology trials (2), the patient's perspective is often dismissed (3). As a result, the patient is seldom provided with an adequate appraisal of the situation and management to be followed, nor with opportunities for discussion and clarification. Indeed, shared decision-making does not seem to characterize current psychiatric practice, unlike in other specialties such as diabetology and cardiovascular medicine. Not surprisingly, a substantial proportion of patients discontinue antidepressant therapy after responding to an initial acute phase of treatment, regardless of the physician's advice (4, 5).

I will analyze the conceptual obstacles that currently hinder decision-making in medicine (with particular focus on antidepressant drugs) and the specific clinical situations where the decisions should be made.

Conceptual Obstacles to Rational Prescribing and Deprescribing

A rational use of drugs depends on the balance of potential benefits and adverse effects applied to the individual patient (6). One problem in achieving such a balance derives from the different sources of information that need to be integrated. Guidelines tend to place emphasis on systematic reviews and meta-analyses of RCTs that are uniquely geared to detecting benefits (7). Observational studies tend to be considered to have less validity, despite evidence that calls such a view into question (7). Appraisal of adverse effects relies primarily on observational studies and data from routine clinical practice, and may not emerge from RCTs, unless these effects occur early in treatment and are specifically investigated (6, 7).

In the current characterization of evidence-based medicine (EBM), which is quite different from its original purposes (8), there is excessive reliance on RCTs and meta-analyses that are not intended to answer questions about the treatment of individual patients (8, 9). The results of RCTs may show the comparative efficacy of treatments for the average randomized patient, but not for those whose characteristics—such as severity of symptoms, comorbidity, and other clinical features—depart from standard presentations (8, 9). Feinstein (10) compared meta-analyses to the alchemy that existed before modern scientific chemistry. The analogy was the hope to convert existing things into something better (changing base metals into gold) and the work with material that was heterogeneous and poorly identified. Indeed, meta-analyses often include highly heterogeneous studies and ascribe conflicting results to random variability, whereas different outcomes may reflect different patient populations, enrollment, and protocol characteristics (8, 11). Not surprisingly, the results of meta-analyses often serve vested interests (8) and are of limited usefulness for informing patient care (12).

EBM does not represent the scientific approach to medicine: it is only a restrictive interpretation of the scientific approach to clinical practice (8). Such an approach is in need of integration in decision analysis. Horwitz et al. (13) developed a method of clinical inquiry within RCTs that can enhance the applicability of results to clinical decision-making. Reanalyzing the Beta-Blocker Heart Attack Trial, they found that propranolol reduced the risk of dying for the "average" patient who survived an acute myocardial infarction, whereas it was harmful in a subgroup characterized by specific co-therapy histories. If we accept the possibility that a treatment which is helpful on average may be ineffective in some and even harmful in someone else, we may learn that a given therapy may not be of value for a particular class or subgroup of subjects who are defined in terms of more detailed (compared to the RCT eligibility criteria) specifications of clinical conditions (13). Richardson and Doster (14) have suggested consideration of three dimensions in the process of evidence-based decision-making: *potential benefits* of the therapeutic option, *responsiveness* to the treatment option, and *vulnerability* to the adverse effects of treatment. EBM is focused on the potential benefits of therapy in relation to the baseline risk, but it is likely to neglect the other two dimensions. Approaching the individual patient, the clinician needs to have a clear account of the potential benefits of a specific treatment, as well as of the predictors of responsiveness, and of the potential adverse events that may be triggered by the therapeutic act (14–16). The achievement of such a balance is hindered by the difficult integration of different sources of information, particularly when, as in the case of antidepressant discontinuation, there is widespread unawareness of the events related to it (17).

Clinical Situations

Regardless of the source of the initiative (patient or prescriber), there are specific circumstances that may determine the need for discontinuing a certain antidepressant medication. I will mention here what I regard as the most common and troublesome, yet the list is not by any means exhaustive. In most of the cases, the decision of interrupting antidepressants should of course be weighed against the risks of leaving depression untreated.

Medical Side Effects

Long-term treatment with newer-generation antidepressant medications, such as SSRIs and SNRIs, may cause important medical side effects (e.g., gastrointestinal symptoms, weight gain, cardiovascular problems, bleeding) (18) which may mandate discontinuation and close medical monitoring (Box 5.1). Unlike TCAs, which cause side effects (e.g., dry mouth, constipation) mainly at the beginning of treatment, with a tendency to decrease as time goes by, newer-generation antidepressants often display their most troublesome side effects after several months of therapy (18). Some of these effects, such as the delayed emergence of weight gain, may be explained by the oppositional model of tolerance I described in the previous chapter, as indicated by a prospective population-based study (19). Indeed, it has been suggested that an increase in exposure to antidepressant drugs may be a driving force for the obesity pandemic (20). In other cases, certain side effects, such as the gastric symptomatology associated with the use of SSRIs and SNRIs, occur at the beginning of treatment and yield a cumulative toxicity over its course (18). The occurrence of such disturbances may initiate cascade iatrogenesis and may require proton pump inhibitors, that may be associated with the risk of major depressive disorder (21). Other types of medical side effects, such as the cardiovascular ones (QT interval prolongation, basal heart rate and heart rate variability, hypertension, orthostatic hypotension) may

---

Box 5.1 Main Medical Adverse Events Related to the Use of Newer-Generation Antidepressant Medications

- gastrointestinal (nausea, vomiting, bleeding)
- hepatotoxicity
- hypersensitivity reactions (skin and vascular)
- weight gain and metabolic disturbances
- cardiovascular
- genitourinary (retention, incontinence)
- hyponatremia
- osteoporosis and liability to fractures
- bleeding
- ophthalmic (glaucoma, cataract)
- central nervous system (headache, lowering of seizure threshold, extrapyramidal side effects, liability to stroke)

have a variable onset during treatment (18, 22). Contrary to expectations, newer-generation antidepressants have not been found to be better than TCAs in terms of mortality related to cardiovascular events (22).

Medical side effects may subside with discontinuation of the anti-depressant medication, as the following case indicates. Other times, medical side effects persist after antidepressant discontinuation, which raises the question of a link with a persistent postwithdrawal medical disorder.

Esther is a 68-year-old housewife who was prescribed venlafaxine (75 mg/day) after the death of her husband, even though she did not present with a major depressive disorder but only with an understandable grief reaction. Shortly after the prescription of venlafaxine, her blood pressure (until then well managed by a diuretic) became difficult to control. She was on two additional anti-hypertensive medications and yet her blood pressure was poorly controlled at the time of my assessment. She also presented with low mood, anxiety, and agitation. I thus decided to taper and discontinue venlafaxine, since it is linked to hypertension (18) and was not effective, and substituted it with clonazepam (0.5 mg twice a day). Esther did not have problems in tapering and discontinuing venlafaxine, and responded well to clonazepam. Her blood pressure went down and she achieved satisfactory control with the use of diuretic only.

Pregnancy and Breastfeeding

There is increasing literature on the potential harmful effects of anti-depressant medications during pregnancy, including birth defects and withdrawal syndromes in the neonates (18). Antidepressant drugs are also transmitted to the child during lactation (18). The request of discontinuing antidepressant medications may come from the patient herself, who has read about these harmful effects on the internet. In the most favorable circumstances, it may precede pregnancy ("I plan to get pregnant and I want to get rid of these medications"). Often, however, the request is formulated at various stages of pregnancy. Close coordination with the gynecologist is thus of paramount importance.

Paradoxical Effects and the Switch Into Bipolar Disorder

Switching into hypomania or mania, apathy, onset of suicidality, and deepening of depressed mood, as examined in Chapter 3, may suggest the necessity of discontinuing antidepressant medications.

Lack or Loss of Efficacy

A specific antidepressant drug may not be effective from the very beginning, despite adequate doses and duration of the trial, or may lose its effectiveness after a certain period, as described in Chapter 3. Lack of efficacy may also take place with an antidepressant that was previously effective (resistance).

Unclear Reasons for Initial Prescription and Automatic Prolongation of Treatment

Antidepressant medications are often prescribed without clear psychiatric indications, when the person is demoralized and/or under stress, and their use may be prolonged for years (23), as I have already described in several clinical vignettes in the previous chapters. In such cases, the clinician and the patient may wish to verify the usefulness of treatment prolongation.

Planned Discontinuation

A physician may prescribe an antidepressant medication and plan to use it for a predetermined time. In the sequential treatment of depression, patients who respond to drug treatment are offered psychotherapy while antidepressant drugs are tapered and discontinued (24). This design has been used in a number of RCTs and was found to produce significant benefits (24, 25). Antidepressant drug continuation was not found to be associated with significant advantages compared to planned discontinuation (24, 25).

Improved Clinical Conditions

A patient who takes antidepressant medications for a mood or anxiety disorder may get better; he or she may request that the drug is discontinued. Another situation may concern an improvement that is secondary to the addition of psychotherapy to the treatment regimen, as was found to be the case in the study where SSRIs were discontinued after behavioral treatment of panic disorder (26).

Patient Preference

This is an issue that is of primary importance, particularly in a setting characterized by shared decision-making. If a patient wishes to have his/her antidepressant medication tapered and discontinued, and the request appears to be reasonable, it is certainly preferable to have the clinician monitoring the process, rather than letting the patient do this by himself/herself. Patients may express the wish to stop antidepressant drugs before they exert their full effects (which takes at least 4–6 weeks), or at a very unsuitable time, or for side effects that can be expected and are likely to wane. Recently, a patient who was doing well on antidepressants after 5 weeks of treatment asked me whether he could stop them suddenly for a week and then take them again "to see what happens." No matter how odd the requests may be, there should always be time for discussing them.

The Role of Clinical Judgment and Shared Decision-Making

In the previous section, I have examined the main clinical situations where the decision of discontinuing antidepressant medications may be made. These situations are very different from each other and one may wonder whether the same approach may be viable for all. Further, treatment outcome is the cumulative result of the interaction of several classes of variables with a selected treatment: living conditions (e.g., housing, nutrition, work environment, social support), patient characteristics (e.g., age, sex, genetic, general health conditions, personality, well-being), illness features and previous therapeutic experience, self-management, and treatment setting (e.g., physician's attitude and attention, patient's illness behavior) (27). Such variables may be therapeutic or counter-therapeutic. In certain patients, their interactive combination may lead to clinical improvement; in other cases, it may produce no effect; and, in a third group, it may lead to worsening of the condition (13).

This multifactorial framework also applies to the therapeutic decision of discontinuing a medication (Figure 5.1). The term "deprescribing" is an understandable reaction to the overprescribing that has occurred in recent years (1), yet it conveys the idea that you are simply subtracting something, with the ensuing sense of vulnerability, instead of substituting one therapeutic ingredient with another.

As Gordon Guyatt (one of the developers of EBM) remarks, there is no single right decision in a specific clinical situation and one should evaluate the potential harms and risks of each therapeutic act (28). Indeed, the model of EBM was originally articulated in a way that high-lighted the many sources of knowledge and how they could be integrated with judgment in the shared decisions for the care of the whole person

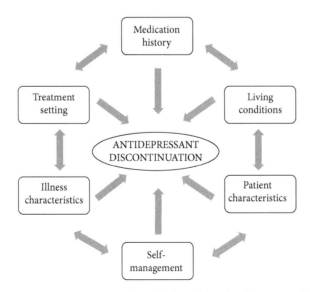

Figure 5.1 Interacting Therapeutic Variables Affecting Treatment Outcome

(29). However, in the following years, vested interests and a lack of familiarity with clinical issues conveyed the message that there is only one option for the treatment of a specific condition. The physician who adheres to guidelines is convinced to apply the best evidence and to be "scientific," and is not aware that he/she is simply guided to see problems in a certain way, to treat the average instead of the individual patient, and to follow the pseudoscience of manipulated meta-analyses (8). In the same vein, the restrictive ideology that characterizes a prevalent reductionist practice of EBM leads the clinician to disregard "non-specific" ingredients as optional and uninfluential, often referring to the fact that "there is no evidence they work," against the clinical awareness that it is the sum of positive ingredients (incremental care) that often leads to improvement in practice (27).

The clinician needs to have a clear account of the potential benefits of a specific treatment, as well as of the predictors of responsiveness, and of the potential adverse events that may be triggered by the therapeutic act (8, 28, 29). Clinical judgment still has the major importance it always had in patient care, as the method of applying the available evidence to the individual case. Engel (30) identified the key characteristic of clinical science in its explicit attention to humanness, where observation (outerviewing), introspection (inner-viewing), and dialogue (inter-viewing) are the basic methodological triad for clinical assessment and for making patient data truly scientific. In 1967, Alvan Feinstein dedicated a monograph to an analysis of clinical judgment and the reasoning that underlies medical evaluations, such as the appraisal of symptoms, signs, and the timing of individual manifestations (31). Also, there is nothing more than clinical judgment when we are called to evaluate the elements depicted in Figure 5.1.

In their everyday practice, psychiatrists use observation, description, and classification, test explanatory hypotheses, and formulate clinical decisions. In evaluating whether a patient needs admission to the hospital (or can be discharged from it), in deciding whether a patient needs treatment (and in that case, what type), and in planning the schedule of follow-up visits or interventions, the psychiatrist, like any other clinician, uses nothing more than the science of clinical judgment (32). However, such an approach is disdainfully tagged as a dangerous departure from established patterns, instead of the exercise of critical thinking (32).

References

1. Gupta S, Miller R, Cahill JD: Deprescribing in Psychiatry. New York, Oxford University Press, 2019.
2. Fava GA, Tomba E, Bech P: Clinical pharmacopsychology: conceptual foundations and emerging tasks. Psychother Psychosom 2017; 86:134–40.
3. Guy A, Brown M, Lewis S, Horowitz M: The 'patient voice': patients who experience antidepressant withdrawal symptoms are often dismissed, or misdiagnosed with relapse, or a new medical condition. Ther Adv Psychopharmacology 2020 Nov 9; 10:2045125320967183.
4. Simon GE, von Korff M, Heilingestein JH, Revicki DA, Grothams L, Katon W, Wagner EH: Initial antidepressant choice in primary care. JAMA 1996; 275:1897–902.
5. Dunn RL, Donoghue JM, Osminkowski RJ, Stephenson D, Hylan TR: Longitudinal patterns of antidepressant prescribing in primary care in the UK. J Psychopharmacol 1999; 13:136–143.
6. Vanderbroucke JP, Psaty BM: Benefits and risks of drug treatments. How to combine the best evidence on benefits with the best data about adverse effects. JAMA 2008; 300:2417–19.
7. Concato J, Shah N, Horwitz RI: Randomized, controlled trials, observational studies, and the hierarchy of research designs. N Engl J Med 2000; 342:1887–92.
8. Fava GA: Evidence-based medicine was bound to fail. J Clin Epidemiol 2017; 84:3–7.
9. Feinstein AR, Horwitz RI: Problems in the "evidence" of "evidence-based medicine." Am J Med 1997; 103:529–35.
10. Feinstein AR: Meta-analysis: statistical alchemy for the 21st century. J Clin Epidemiol 1995; 48:71–9.
11. Jane-Wit D, Horwitz RI, Concato J: Variation in results from randomized, controlled trials: stochastic or systematic? J Clin Epidemiol 2010; 63:56–63.
12. Concato J, Horwitz RI: Limited usefulness of meta-analysis for informing patient care. Psychother Psychosom 2019; 88:257–62.
13. Horwitz RI, Singer BH, Makuch RW, Viscoli CM: Can treatment that is helpful on average be harmful to some patients? J Clin Epidemiol 1996; 49:395–400.
14. Richardson WS, Doster LM: Comorbidity and multimorbidity need to be placed in the context of a framework of risk, responsiveness, and vulnerability. J Clin Epidemiol 2014; 67:244–6.
15. Vanderbroucke JP, Psaty BM: Benefits and risks of drug treatments. How to combine the best evidence on benefits with the best data about adverse effects. JAMA 2008; 300:2417–19.
16. Fava GA: Rational use of antidepressant drugs. Psychother Psychosom 2014; 83:197–204.
17. Fava GA, Belaise C: Discontinuing antidepressant drugs. Psychother Psychosom 2018; 87:257–67.
18. Carvalho AF, Sharma MS, Brunoni AR, Vieta E, Fava GA: The safety, tolerability and risks associated with the use of newer generation antidepressant drugs. Psychother Psychosom 2016; 85:270–88.

19. Patten SB, Williams JV, Lavorato DH, Brown L, McLaren L, Eliasziw M: Major depression, antidepressant medication and the risk of obesity. Psychother Psychosom 2009; 78:182–6.
20. Lee SH, Paz-Filho G, Matronardi C, Licinio J, Wong MI: Is increased antidepressant exposure a contributory factor to the obesity pandemic? Transl Psychiatry 2016; 6:e759.
21. Huang WS, Bai YM, Hsu JW, Huang KL, Tsai CF, Su TP, Li CT, Lin WC, Tsai SJ, Pan TL, Chen TJ, Chen MH: Use of proton pump inhibitors and risk of major depressive disorder. Psychother Psychosom 2018; 87:62–4.
22. Maslej MM, Bolker BM, Russell MJ, Eaton K, Durisko Z, Hollon SD, Swanson GM, Thomson JA, Mulsant BH, Andrews PW: The mortality and myocardial effects of antidepressants are moderated by pre-existing cardiovascular disease. Psychother Psychosom 2017; 86:268–82.
23. Huijbregts KM, Hoogendoorn AW, Slottje P, van Balkom AJLM, Batelaan NM: Long-term and short-term antidepressant use in general practice. Psychother Psychosom 2017; 86:362–9.
24. Guidi J, Tomba E, Fava GA: The sequential integration of pharmacotherapy and psychotherapy in the treatment of major depressive disorder: a meta-analysis of the sequential model and a critical review of the literature. Am J Psychiatry 2016; 173:128–37.
25. Guidi J, Fava GA: Sequential combination of pharmacotherapy and psychotherapy in major depressive disorder: a systematic review and meta-analysis. JAMA Psychiatry 2021; 78:261-9.
26. Fava GA, Bernardi M, Tomba E, Rafanelli C: Effects of gradual discontinuation of selective serotonin reuptake inhibitors in panic disorder with agoraphobia. Int J Neuropsychopharmacol 2007; 10:835–8.
27. Fava GA, Guidi J, Rafanelli C, Rickels K: The clinical inadequacy of the placebo model and the development of an alternative conceptual framework. Psychother Psychosom. 2017; 86:332–40.
28. Guyatt G: EBM has not only called out the problems but offered solutions. J Clin Epidemiol 2017; 84:8–10.
29. Richardson WS: The practice of evidence-base medicine involves the care of the whole persons. J Clin Epidemiol 2017; 84:18–21.
30. Engel GL: How much longer must medicine's science be bound by a seventeenth century world view? Psychother Psychosom 1992; 57:3–16.
31. Feinstein AR: Clinical Judgment. Baltimore, Williams & Wilkins, 1967.
32. Fava GA: Clinical judgment in psychiatry: requiem or reveille? Nord J Psychiatry 2013; 67:1–10.

6

The Setting of Guided Antidepressant Discontinuation

I have accumulated most of my clinical experience with discontinuing antidepressant medications in a clinical setting that has some specific characteristics—an Affective Disorders Program that I established in Northern Italy in the early nineties for applying the sequential model to the treatment of both mood and anxiety disorders (1). The sequential model comprises the consecutive application of two forms of treatment: psychotherapy after pharmacotherapy, pharmacotherapy after psychotherapy, or the sequential use of two psychotherapeutic or pharmacological strategies (1). It is an intensive, two-stage approach, which derives from the awareness that one course of treatment with a specific intervention (whether pharmacotherapy or psychotherapy) is unlikely to solve the affective disturbances of patients, both in research and clinical practice settings. The Affective Disorders Program is run by the combined efforts of psychiatrists, internists, and clinical psychologists. The initial activities soon expanded to those of a special problems outpatient clinic, geared to trying to provide an answer to unusual and/or complicated and/or treatment-resistant cases. Referral sources may be primary care physicians and other medical specialists, clinical psychologists, psychiatrists, or patients themselves.

As the psychiatrist providing the initial evaluation (as well as subsequent pharmacological treatment in most of the cases, and psychotherapy in selected cases), I was confronted with the problems caused by discontinuation of antidepressant drugs. For instance, psychologists referred patients with remitted anxiety disorders (e.g., panic and phobias) as a result of psychological treatments, who had trouble getting off their medications (2). Or primary care physicians, who had prescribed mostly SSRIs and SNRIs to their patients, and were unable to find a way to discontinue these medications, asked for help. Or colleagues from all over the country, who self-prescribed antidepressants, wanted to know the trick for getting off these drugs. My very extensive clinical experience (hundreds of cases) was, as with the rest of my clinical encounters, characterized by high severity, persistence, resistance, and complications of symptomatology. Obviously, the patient who did not encounter problems in discontinuing his or her antidepressant was unlikely to come to us. My practice is also biased toward another characteristic: in almost all cases concerned with discontinuation problems, the initial prescription did not come from me (it would have been rather difficult since I seldom prescribe SSRIs, and I have never prescribed a SNRI). I thus learned how important (and difficult) is the medication history, as I will discuss in the next chapter. Over the years, I gained insight on the fact that getting off an antidepressant medication is often more complicated and technical than getting on, that a patient may be exempt from withdrawal but not from relapse, and that the structure of the sequential model of treatment was absolutely necessary for providing adequate support to the patient who wanted to stop taking antidepressants. Indeed, I argue that discontinuation of antidepressants that is performed without medical consultation and adequate psychotherapeutic support entails substantial risks for the patient and is often bound to fail. An alternative could be clinical services specifically addressing the discontinuation of psychotropic drugs.

I will outline here the model provided by our Affective Disorders Program and another type of service initiated by Fiammetta Cosci at the University of Florence, as examples of clinical settings geared to the discontinuation of antidepressant medications.

A New Model of Outpatient Clinic for Affective Disorders

I will discuss the staffing, functioning, and modalities of integration of the basic operational unit of the outpatient clinic, which could be multiplied according to the number and needs of the patients served (3). The basic unit includes a psychiatrist, an internist, and four psychotherapists (in our case clinical psychologists). The psychiatrist should have an adequate background both in psychopharmacology and psychotherapy. Experience in performing psychotherapy is essential—whether or not the psychiatrist will provide it in the clinic—since referral to psychotherapy requires a deep understanding of the indications and contraindications of the psychotherapeutic technique that is suggested. The internist should be able to provide specialized medical evaluation, especially of endocrine and cardiovascular problems, and be familiar with the use of psychotropic drugs. Psychotherapists may have different levels of experience and training in evidence-based psychotherapeutic strategies, such as cognitive-behavioral therapy (CBT), with particular emphasis on supervising self-therapy approaches (e.g., exposure homework) and on the role of the patient in the process of recovery, including diet and exercise (3). The functioning of the clinic requires close coordination of the team members, with repeated psychiatric assessments and medical evaluation (3).

Psychiatric Assessment

In the current clinic model, which is endorsed in many contexts worldwide, a diagnosis and treatment plan are usually developed after a single initial visit and tend to be followed in the subsequent months or years without any additional time for re-evaluation. This approach is based on a unidimensional, cross-sectional view of the disorder, with the implicit assumption that the illness does not evolve and the diagnosis does not change over time (3). For instance, it is not uncommon for apparently clear-cut unipolar major depression to be re-diagnosed as bipolar disorder, because the prodromes of the manic episode were overlooked or masked at the initial assessment. Accurate diagnosis and effective treatment often depend on repeated assessments, but in standard clinic settings there is insufficient time available to the prescriber for this process (3). Even if the therapist had sufficient expertise to refine the diagnosis, time and structure are not available for a collaborative discussion with the prescriber for comprehensive reconsideration.

Medical Evaluation

Between 20% and 50% of psychiatric patients have active medical illnesses (4, 5), and psychiatric medications such as antidepressant drugs may pose additional medical risks (6). A full understanding of the patient's medical condition is important not only to clarify psychiatric symptoms, but also to determine the need for general medical care and to choose psychiatric treatments that do not interact adversely with the medical illness and its treatment. It is axiomatic that a medical diagnosis depends on a careful history and physical examination, with laboratory investigations as indicated (4, 7). Yet, such evaluations are rarely performed in the clinic setting by psychiatrists or anyone else (8).

Repeated psychiatric assessments and medical evaluation are the mainstay of antidepressant discontinuation. It should also be noted that it is not always easy to obtain adequate collaboration from medical colleagues. I once contacted a cardiologist treating a patient with anticoagulant therapy, alerting him that I was going to taper and discontinue sertraline (prescribed without any valid reason) and that therapy might need adjustments. His resentful reply stated that there was no interaction as far as he knew (and he knew very little, I must say) and that I should mind my own business. My mentor Robert Kellner used to say that the most difficult part of medicine was dealing with colleagues, not patients. Having an internist who has an understanding of the problems we encounter in psychiatry, including those linked to discontinuation of psychotropic drugs, is a considerable advantage. Let us consider the case of Esther, described in the previous chapter, who had her hypertension worsened by venlafaxine. Anti-hypertensive treatment had to be adjusted after discontinuation of venlafaxine—something that a psychiatrist would not be generally comfortable with. Or let us think of a patient on a SSRI who takes protein pump inhibitors, with limited results, for gastric problems (which may be SSRI-induced): an internist is needed for reassessing the need for protein pump inhibitors once the SSRI is discontinued.

The Clinical Pharmacopsychology Service

In the past two decades, websites have been an invaluable source of support for patients attempting to discontinue antidepressant medications or suffering from persistent postwithdrawal disorders (9, 10). Indeed, the web is the main source of referral to a new type of clinical service that has recently been launched (11). Its name, clinical pharmacopsychology service, derives from a new area of clinical psychology that is concerned with the psychological effects of medications (11, 12). The domains of clinical pharmacopsychology encompass the clinical benefits of psychotropic drugs, the characteristics that predict responsiveness to treatment, the vulnerabilities induced by treatment (side effects, behavioral toxicity, iatrogenic comorbidity), and the interactions between drug treatment and psychological variables. Its aim is to provide a comprehensive assessment of the clinical changes that are concerned with the pharmacopsychometric triangle introduced by Per Bech (13):

1. wanted and expected treatment effects;
2. treatment-induced unwanted side effects;
3. patient's own personal experience of a change in terms of well-being and/or quality of life.

The assessment that is performed in the service, which heavily relies on telemedicine and internet interventions, results from a multidisciplinary effort (psychiatrists, clinical psychologists, internists) similar to the model of the Affective Disorders Program I described in the previous section.

Looking for a Place in Healthcare

A primary care physician looked for my advice. He had self-prescribed paroxetine 20 mg/day at a time when he was going through a painful divorce:

> I had seen many patients of mine getting a lot of benefit from this medication and I thought that I could be one of those. It actually helped: I felt some relief and I experienced some sound sleep after several weeks. But my problems with my former wife were not over and trying to save our children from our fight was not easy. So I thought I better keep on taking paroxetine, as a sort of protection. After a couple of years things were looking up a bit and I decided it was time to quit. I knew I had to do

it gradually, so I split the 20 mg tablet. A nightmare: a flare up of somatic symptoms with total loss of concentration (I could not even work as a doctor). I went back to the original dose and things got better. I remembered that this happened also to some patients of mine; I had looked for advice to a couple of psychiatrists I was familiar with for a few patients who had problems similar to mine, and they just suggested to me that those patients had simply to go back to the medications they took before. So I thought that maybe I was not ready and waited a few months. But the same happened again. I checked again with one of the two psychiatrists and she said "You are simply experiencing a relapse. Keep on taking your tablet." I knew it was not true: relapse of what? I had never experienced the type of depression I had seen in my patients. I realized I was in a no man's land, that I had a disease, but there was no place to go. As a primary care physician I became quite good in referring my patients to proper specialist care. But I could not do anything for myself.

This account reminded me of what George Engel had written in one of his most important papers, "A unified concept of health and disease," published in 1960 (14).

The traditional attitude toward disease tends in practice to restrict what it categorized as disease to what can be understood or recognized by the physician and/or what he notes can be helped by his intervention. This attitude has plagued medicine throughout its history and still stands in the way of physicians fully appreciating disease as a natural phenomenon. (14, p. 471)

There is currently no place for providing competent healthcare to people who suffer from the consequences of antidepressant tapering and discontinuation. Physicians are not even able, in an environment controlled and shaped by the pharmaceutical industry, to "think iatrogenic" (15).

References

1. Fava GA: Sequential treatment: a new way of integrating pharmacotherapy and psychotherapy. Psychother Psychosom 1999; 68:227–9.
2. Fava GA, Bernardi M, Tomba E, Rafanelli C: Effects of gradual discontinuation of selective serotonin reuptake inhibitors in panic disorder with agoraphobia. Int J Neuropsychopharmacol 2007; 10:835–8.
3. Fava GA, Park SK, Dubovsky SL: The mental health clinic. A new model. World Psychiatry 2008; 7:177–81.
4. Schiffer RB, Klein RF, Sider RC: The Medical Evaluation of Psychiatric Patients. New York, Plenum Press, 1998.
5. Sartorius N, Holt RIG, Maj M (eds): Comorbidity of Mental and Physical Disorders. Basel, Karger, 2015.
6. Carvalho AF, Sharma MS, Brunoni AR, Vieta E, Fava GA: The safety, tolerability and risks associated with the use of newer generation antidepressant drugs. Psychother Psychosom 2016; 85:270–88.
7. Sonino N, Peruzzi P: A psychoneuroendocrinology service. Psychother Psychosom 2009; 78:346–51.
8. McIntyre JS, Romano J: Is there a stethoscope in the house (and is it used?)? Arch Gen Psychiatry 1977; 34:1147–51.
9. Belaise C, Gatti A, Chouinard VA, Chouinard G: Patient online report of selective serotonin reuptake inhibitor (SSRI) induced persistent postwithdrawal anxiety and mood disorders. Psychother Psychosom 2012; 81:386–8.
10. Hengartner MP, Schulthess L, Sorensen A, Framer A: Protracted withdrawal syndrome after stopping antidepressants: a descriptive quantitative analysis of consumer narratives from a large internet forum. Ther Adv Psychopharmacology 2020 Dec 24; 10:2045125320980573.
11. Cosci F, Guidi J, Tomba E, Fava GA: The emerging role of clinical pharmacopsychology. Clin Psychol Eur 2019; 1:35128.
12. Fava GA, Tomba E, Bech P: Clinical pharmacopsychology: conceptual foundations and emerging tasks. Psychother Psychosom 2017; 8:134–40.
13. Bech P: Applied psychometrics in clinical psychiatry. Acta Psychiatr Scand 2009; 120:400–9.
14. Engel GL: A unified concept of health and disease. Perspect Biol Med 1960; 3:459–85.
15. Fava GA, Rafanelli C: Iatrogenic factors in psychopathology. Psychother Psychosom 2019; 88:129–40.

7

The Role of Clinical Assessment

Diagnostic criteria, such as those of the DSM-5 (1), have become the basis for case formulation and treatment. The main emphasis has been given to the standardization of the assessment process leading to diagnostic configuration (2), and many times a drug prescription is the only automatic translation of this clinical process.

Customary clinical taxonomy in psychiatry does not include patterns of symptoms, severity of illness, effects of comorbid conditions, timing of phenomena, rate of progression of illness, responses to previous treatments, and other clinical distinctions that demarcate major prognostic and therapeutic differences among patients who otherwise seem to be deceptively similar since they share the same psychiatric diagnosis (3). Little consideration has been given to the clinical process in psychiatry—that is, how clinical judgment leading to medical decisions is formulated (3).

In 1982, Alvan Feinstein introduced the term "clinimetrics" (4) to indicate a domain concerned with the measurement of clinical issues that do not find room in customary clinical taxonomy. Such issues include the types, severity, and sequence of symptoms; rate of progression in illness (staging); severity of comorbidity; effects of previous treatments; problems of functional capacity; reasons for medical decisions (e.g., treatment choices); and many other aspects of daily life, such as well-being and distress (5, 6). Clinimetric research in psychiatry has yielded important insights as to the role and function of clinical judgment (3) and the enduring effects of previous treatments (7).

In the past two decades, the use of psychotropic medications has dramatically increased: one out of six adults in USA is reported to take psychiatric drugs at least once during a year, and in eight out of 10 cases it is for long-term use (8). Antidepressant drugs lead the ranking of medications (8). This issue is further complicated by the frequent practice of polypharmacy in medicine and psychiatry (9).

Current diagnostic methods in psychiatry (1, 2) refer to patients who are drug-free and do not take the issue of iatrogenic comorbidity into adequate consideration. They are suited for a patient who no longer exists: most of the psychiatric cases that are seen in clinical practice receive some form of psychotropic drug treatment at the time of the first psychiatric or psychological assessment and require evaluation of iatrogenic factors.

Diagnostic criteria in the setting of guided antidepressant medication discontinuation thus need to be integrated by a specific clinimetric approach geared to data gathering, organization of findings, and formulation of treatment plans that is not usually performed in practice. In addition to the customary clinical assessment (2), clinimetric elements related to treatment history and staging, the assessment of current clinical state, macroanalysis, and the monitoring of progress of tapering and discontinuation, will be outlined in this chapter. I argue that such an assessment is necessary for an informed decision on the clinical situations described in Chapter 5. This accurate evaluation is particularly important when the clinician monitoring the choice is not the same person who had prescribed the antidepressant medication.

Treatment History and Staging

In psychiatric and psychological assessment, there is insufficient emphasis on collecting information related to previous treatment. For instance, the Third Edition of the American Psychiatric Association's *Practice Guidelines for the Psychiatric Evaluation of Adults* (2) does mention the importance of reviewing prior psychiatric treatment, either with open-ended questions or with a detailed inquiry about each treatment in sequence. However, it does not provide any specific indication as to the type of information that can be particularly meaningful.

A first crucial point is to collect data about previous treatments with antidepressant medications, not only as to their efficacy but also as to the occurrence of adverse effects, especially phenomena of behavioral toxicity, as suggested in Box 7.1. These questions may take some time, and patients may not have documentation about their previous antidepressant drugs history (e.g., my secretary always reminds patients to bring

---

Box 7.1 Key Questions for Assessing Behavioral Toxicity of Antidepressant Medications

---

1. Which sequence of antidepressant drugs were administered in the past (duration, dosages, adherence)? Particular attention should be given to the concurrent use of medical drugs and to the occurrence of substance misuse.
2. Was there a satisfactory response?
3. Were there any paradoxical effects (e.g., increased depression) with any of these medications or their combinations?
4. Was there any switching to an opposite condition (e.g., hypomania or mania with antidepressant drugs) both during or immediately after treatment?
5. Was there any loss of clinical effects, despite adequate adherence, during long-term antidepressant treatment?
6. Was there any lack of response to a previously effective pharmacological treatment when it was started again after a drug-free period?
7. Has the patient any history of antidepressant drug refractoriness?
8. Did any withdrawal syndromes occur upon tapering and/ or discontinuation of antidepressant drugs? Any persistent postwithdrawal disorders?

---

all medical information, but the success rate is pretty low) or may not remember. Sometimes one needs to recheck information in a subsequent assessment or to get a relative in.

It is very important not to limit information to psychotropic medications, but to extend it to drugs directed to medical conditions which may induce psychiatric syndromes (10), with particular reference to those specifically associated with the onset of depression (11–13), such as corticosteroids, anticonvulsants, oral contraceptives, GnRH agonists, tamoxifen, and interferon. In a large cross-sectional survey (14), use of multiple medications with the potential for depression as an adverse effect was associated with a greater likelihood of concurrent depression. It is also important to collect information about previous experiences, if any, with psychotherapy, because they may affect future indications. The information that is collected with the treatment history lends itself to the use of staging methods.

For a long time, psychiatry had neglected staging as a model to classify the longitudinal development of mental disorders. In 1993, Robert Kellner and I (15) introduced the clinimetric concept of staging in psychiatric classification. Thus, once an index defines the existence of a particular disease state (diagnostic criteria), its seriousness, extent, and longitudinal characteristics need to be evaluated (15, 16). Figure 7.1 outlines the basic classification of the stages of a major depressive disorder. The prodromal phase (stage 1) is characterized by the onset of depressive symptoms, mainly anxiety, irritable mood, anhedonia, and sleep disorders. There is large inter-individual variability in prodromes; however, for a specific patient, different episodes of illness tend to share similar prodromal symptomatology (15, 16). At stage 2, subjects present with the major depressive episode; then a residual phase (stage 3) may occur. Residual symptoms are a strong predictor of relapse (16). Certain prodromal symptoms may be overshadowed by the acute manifestations of the disorder, but persist as residual symptoms and progress to become prodromes of relapse. Detre and Jarecki (17) provided a model for relating prodromal and residual symptomatology in psychiatric illness, defined as the rollback phenomenon: as the illness remits, it progressively recapitulates, even though in reverse order, many of the stages and symptoms that were seen during the time it developed. There is also a temporal relationship between the time of development of a disorder and the duration of the phase of recovery. The rollback phenomenon has been substantiated in mood and anxiety disorders (16). Stage 4 is characterized by chronicity that may be expressed as recurrent depression or double depression (persistent depression interspersed by episodes of major depressive disorder), or by a chronic major depressive episode lasting at least 2 years without interruptions.

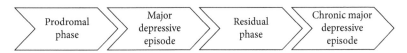

Figure 7.1 The Longitudinal Development (Staging) of Depressive Disorders

Staging also takes into consideration the response of the disease to specific therapies, with particular reference to treatment resistance (16), which may be caused by iatrogenic manifestations of behavioral toxicity (18). These latter manifestations may also be viewed in light of the oppositional model of tolerance and classified according to staging method (Box 7.2) (18). Even though there are no published data about it, it is conceivable that occurrence of one or more of the events related to behavioral toxicity (stages 1–4 of Box 7.2) may be associated with the risk of

---

Box 7.2 Manifestations of Oppositional Tolerance in Current and/or Previous Depressive Episodes According to a Staging Method*

STAGE 0: No occurrence of the following events:

1. paradoxical effects (i.e., increased depression with antidepressants)
2. switching to hypomania or mania while on antidepressants
3. loss of clinical effect of antidepressants, despite adequate adherence
4. lack of response to a previously effective antidepressant treatment when it was started again after a drug-free period
5. withdrawal syndrome after tapering and/or switching and/or discontinuation of an antidepressant**
6. persistent postwithdrawal disorder after discontinuation of an antidepressant**

STAGE 1: Occurrence of one of the above events
STAGE 2: Occurrence of two of the above events
STAGE 3: Occurrence of three of the above events
STAGE 4: Occurrence of four or more of the above events

* Modified from reference 18
** According to Cosci and Chouinard (19)

Source data from Fava GA, Cosci F, Guidi J, Rafanelli C: The deceptive manifestations of treatment resistance in depression. Psychother Psychosom 2020; 89:265–73.

Cosci F, Chouinard G: Acute and persistent withdrawal syndromes following discontinuation of psychotropic medications. Psychother Psychosom 2020; 89:283–306.

developing withdrawal syndromes during tapering or after discontinuation of antidepressant medications. Indeed, my clinical experience would support such an association.

Assessment of the Current Condition and Macroanalysis

The DSM-5 (1) has major limitations in the assessment of the current condition of the patient for whom a discontinuation of antidepressant medications is considered. One drawback is the flat, cross-sectional view of disorders that DSM-5 provides (1). When assessing a patient who is in an apparent stable condition and is taking antidepressant medications, attention should be paid to the presence and characteristics of residual symptomatology, defined as the persistence of symptoms and signs despite apparent remission or recovery (20–22). Such symptoms are the rule after completion of drug or psychotherapeutic treatment of depression. It is thus necessary to perform a complete evaluation of a patient's symptomatology as to both depressive and anxiety symptoms. Since residual symptoms are a strong predictor of relapse (20–22), the presence of substantial residual symptomatology, despite apparent remission, should alert the clinician to the risks entailed by treatment discontinuation and calls for a sequential model of treatment—that is, discontinuation can be carried out only during or after a course of psychotherapy addressing residual symptomatology (20–22). The importance of staging in providing a configuration to symptoms becomes manifest. One thing is the presence of a limited number of depressive symptoms—not sufficient to formulate the diagnosis of a major depressive episode—in patients who are drug-free. Another thing is the presence of the same symptoms in patients undergoing long-term antidepressant treatment. Should we evaluate those symptoms simply on the basis of cross-sectional current symptomatology regardless of treatment status, as the DSM-5 (1) would indicate, or taking a longitudinal perspective including current drug treatment using staging methods (15, 16)?

A further limitation of the DSM-5 (1) is the lack of reference to psychosocial and environmental problems, unlike in previous editions, such as in the DSM-IV (23), where they were coded in the fourth axis. Stressful life circumstances, occupational and financial problems, family and interpersonal frictions are examples. Such an omission is particularly serious in evaluating an apparently recovered patient still taking antidepressant treatment, because of the strong link between life events and depressive relapse (24). Fortunately, a method for evaluating the stressfulness of the patient's environment is available and is represented by the diagnosis of allostatic overload (25). Allostatic load refers to the cumulative burden of chronic stress and life events (26, 27). It involves the interaction of different physiological systems at varying degrees of activity. When environmental challenges exceed the individual ability to cope, then allostatic overload ensues (25, 27). In addition to being associated with deranged biomarkers, allostatic load is identified by clinimetric criteria that are presented in Box 7.3. Such a diagnosis is part of the Diagnostic Criteria for Psychosomatic Research (DCPR) (28).

Box 7.3 Clinical Criteria for Allostatic Overload (A Through B Required)*

Criterion A   The presence of a current source of distress in the form of recent life events and/or chronic stress; the stressor is judged to tax or exceed the individual coping skills when its full nature and circumstances are evaluated.

Criterion B   The stressor is associated with one or more of the following features, which have occurred within 6 months after the onset of the stressor:

1. at least two of the following symptoms (difficulty falling asleep, restless sleep, early morning awakening, lack of energy, dizziness, generalized anxiety, irritability, sadness, demoralization);
2. significant impairment in social or occupational functioning;
3. significant impairment in environmental mastery (feeling overwhelmed by the demands of everyday life).

* Modified from reference 25

Source data from Fava GA, McEwen BS, Guidi J, Gostoli S, Offidani E, Sonino N: Clinical characterization of allostatic overload. Psychoneuroendocrinology 2019; 108:94–101.

A final limitation of the DSM-5 is the lack of reference to psychological well-being. Dimensions such as environmental mastery, personal growth, purpose in life, autonomy, self-acceptance, and positive relations with others were found to affect vulnerability to life adversities and the complex balance between positive and negative affect in mood and anxiety disorders (29). Euthymia is generally conceived in negative terms (absence of psychiatric disorders), yet it may also indicate a transdiagnostic construct where lack of mood disturbances is associated with positive affect and psychological well-being (flexibility, consistency, and resilience) (30). Specific strategies for the assessment of euthymia are available, including both observer- and self-rated instruments that may be applied within a clinimetric framework (29), as I am going to describe in Chapter 11.

When Feinstein (31) introduced the concept of comorbidity, he referred to any "additional co-existing ailment" separate from the primary disease, even in the case that this secondary phenomenon does not qualify as a disease per se. Indeed, in clinical medicine, the many methods that are available for measuring comorbidity are not limited to disease entities (32). On the contrary, in psychiatry there is still the tendency to rely exclusively on diagnostic criteria and psychiatric symptoms, excluding other information related, for instance, to stress and impairment (3).

In clinical psychology, Emmelkamp et al. (33) introduced the concept of macroanalysis (i.e., a relationship between co-occurring syndromes and problems is established on the basis of where treatment should commence in the first place). This model has been revised and expanded to incorporate the full spectrum of comorbidities that is covered by Feinstein's concept of comorbidity (31), including psychosocial problems, functional impairments, and treatment history (iatrogenic comorbidity) (3, 25). Nicoletta Sonino, Thomas Wise, and I have also applied macroanalysis to assessing the relationship between medical and psychological variables (34). Macroanalysis starts from the assumption that, in most cases, there are functional relationships with other more or less clearly defined problem areas and that the targets of treatment may vary during the course of disturbances. An example of macroanalysis is provided by the following case.

Charles is a 47-year-old clerk who was referred to us for treatment-resistant depression, as an inadequate response to two consecutive trials with antidepressant medications (first paroxetine and then venlafaxine), at therapeutic doses and for an adequate time (35). Careful and thorough interviewing, following the lines that have been previously described, disclosed long-standing work situational social anxiety (which was not sufficient for a DSM diagnosis (1), but led him to avoid important opportunities for improving his job) and marital crisis (due to the patient's perfectionism). Depressed mood was present, but it was not accompanied by other symptoms that characterize a major depressive disorder (1). Charles displayed an initial good response to paroxetine, but it subsided after 3 months of treatment. His primary care physician then switched him to venlafaxine, this time with modest results (hence the referral to us). The transition from paroxetine to venlafaxine was gradual, but was associated with a withdrawal syndrome. Macroanalysis lends itself to the full use of clinical judgment. I could place the syndromes and symptoms of comorbidity into a hierarchy by considering also the patient's needs (Figure 7.2). Some clinical phenomena (loss of clinical efficacy and withdrawal syndrome in the transition between paroxetine and venlafaxine) were consistent with the oppositional model of tolerance (see Chapter 4). I thus inserted "iatrogenic comorbidity" in the initial macroanalysis. As a result, the patient was at high risk of withdrawal syndrome with venlafaxine discontinuation (Box 7.2, stage 2) and I did not want to start treatment by changing the medication. I gave priority to CBT, primarily addressed to social fears, keeping venlafaxine therapy. Further steps had to be planned at the second (post-CBT) assessment (Figure 7.3). CBT was quite effective in reducing social anxiety and yielded some improvement in the work situation, with ensuing amelioration of mood. After the

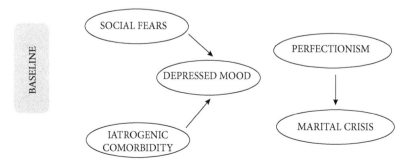

Figure 7.2 Baseline Assessment According to Macroanalysis

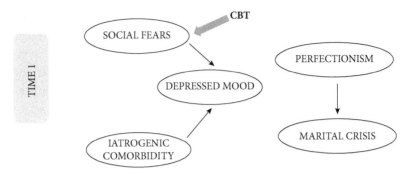

Figure 7.3 Cognitive-Behavioral Therapy (CBT) (Time 1)

second assessment, I decided to start tapering venlafaxine, with the aim of discontinuing it, and to use WBT (36), targeted to perfectionism and marital crisis (Figure 7.4). Indeed, these latter improved after WBT, with techniques emphasizing the negative effects of excessive preoccupation for order and precision, leading to a chronic malaise and communicative difficulties with the partner. In tapering venlafaxine during the course of WBT, there were withdrawal symptoms; however, the patient could successfully handle these. At the third assessment (post-WBT), Charles was drug-free. He still had mild symptoms related to social anxiety and perfectionism, but his improved conditions at work and in the family appeared to be more important.

If the clinical decision of tackling one syndrome may be taken during the initial assessment, the subsequent steps of macroanalysis require a

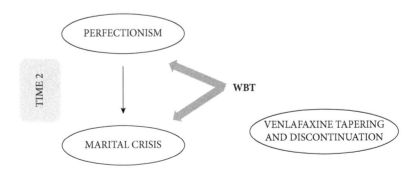

Figure 7.4 Well-Being Therapy (WBT) After the Second Assessment (Time 2)

reassessment after the first line of treatment has terminated. The hierarchical organization that is chosen may depend on a variety of factors (urgency, availability of treatment tools, etc.) that include also the patient's preferences and priorities. Macroanalysis is not only a tool for the therapist, but can also be used to inform the patient about the relationships between different problem areas, to support shared decision-making, and to motivate the patient for changing.

Macroanalysis also requires reference to the staging method, whereby a disorder is characterized according to seriousness, extension, and longitudinal development (15, 16), in addition to iatrogenic comorbidity (18). For instance, certain psychotherapeutic strategies can be deferred to a residual stage of depression, when state-dependent learning has been improved by use of antidepressant drugs (22). The planning of treatment thus requires determination of the symptomatic target of the first-line approach (e.g., pharmacotherapy) and tentative identification of other areas of concern to be addressed by subsequent treatment (e.g., psychotherapy).

Assessing Affective and Withdrawal Symptoms During Tapering and After Discontinuation of Antidepressant Drugs

There should be clear definitions of "relapse/recurrence," "new withdrawal symptoms," "rebound," and "persistent postwithdrawal disorder," according to the criteria we described in Chapter 2 (19, 37): relapse and recurrence are the gradual return of the original symptoms at the same intensity as before treatment, entailing a return of the same episode and a new episode of illness, respectively; new withdrawal symptoms are withdrawal symptoms that are new and not part of the patient's original illness (see Box 2.2, p. 16); rebound symptoms are a rapid return of the patient's original symptoms at a greater intensity than before treatment; persistent postwithdrawal disorder consists of protracted withdrawal symptoms and/or a return of the original symptoms at a greater intensity and/or appearance of new symptoms/disorders that were not present before (see Box 2.3, p. 17). The clinician should be familiar with and investigate withdrawal symptoms that are listed in Box 2.1 (see p. 13). If some open-ended questions may start the exploration, the systematic use of the checklist provided in Box 7.1 is suggested. Clinimetric indices such as the Discontinuation-Emergent Signs and Symptoms (DESS) questionnaire (38) may be very helpful. A semi-structured research interview for applying Chouinard's diagnostic criteria has also been developed (39). A problem concerning new withdrawal symptoms is that they are often general and non-specific. "Brain zaps" (sensations perceived as electrical flashes that occur inside the brain) are probably the most specific, and yet a poorly understood, assessed, and appreciated disturbance (40). The term emerged on internet discussions; other definitions by patients are "electric shock sensations" and "buzz sensations" (40). In my clinical experience, that is confirmed by internet surveys (40), these symptoms are rather disabling. They may subside after a few weeks, but they may also continue for months or years and become part of a persistent postwithdrawal disorder (see, for instance, the case of Emma in Chapter 3).

Withdrawal symptoms can easily be misinterpreted as signs of relapse. Indeed, trial designs that assess the effects of discontinuing antidepressant drugs for inferring efficacy (i.e., a significant increase in depressive symptoms in the patients whose medications are discontinued and switched to placebo compared to those who continue with treatment) are flawed by the lack of consideration and proper assessment of withdrawal events (41–43). The clinical difficulty is increased by the fact that relapse and withdrawal syndromes may coexist. Discriminating issues may be as follows:

1. It is important to have a history of illness progression in the individual patients, since prodromal symptoms of relapse tend to mirror those of the initial episode both in mood (20) and anxiety (16) disorders, and to investigate prodromal symptoms when patients are in remission, to facilitate a better recall (20). Use of observer rating scales, such as Paykel's Clinical Interview for Depression (44), the most sensitive and accurate version of the Hamilton Depression Rating Scale (45), may also help with detection and discrimination of symptoms (20).

2. Withdrawal symptoms are new symptoms that were not part of the patient's symptomatology and, in many cases, do not pertain to depressive disturbances (19, 37).

3. In depression, withdrawal symptoms are likely to have an early onset, while recurrent symptoms generally present with a gradual return (20). This is only a general tendency, however, and not a rule; these patterns do not apply in anxiety disorders.

4. Withdrawal symptoms have a tendency to wane with time (unless they develop into persistent withdrawal disorders), whereas the opposite trend occurs with prodromal symptoms of relapse (16, 20).

However, all these subtle issues in differential diagnosis may break under the wall represented by the psychiatrist who has been brainwashed by pharmaceutical propaganda.

Claire is a 37-year-old secretary who was successfully treated for an episode of major depression with venlafaxine 75 mg/day by a young psychiatrist working in a mental health center. After one year of treatment, the drug was tapered and discontinued. A few days after stopping, the patient reported insomnia, agitation, various somatic symptoms, and "brain zaps." The psychiatrist told her it was a depressive relapse and that venlafaxine had to be reinstituted. Claire was, however, doubtful ("I do not feel depressed") and so was her primary care physician, who asked me for urgent consultation. The withdrawal nature of symptoms was evident. I called the young psychiatrist, who refused to entertain this possibility ("I never heard of withdrawal reactions with antidepressants during my residency training and in subsequent meetings") and was not interested in reading literature that was offered.

A final assessment strategy that is currently neglected involves mental pain, characterized by a persistent and irreversible feeling of internal and not localized pain, a sense of emptiness, or a lack of meaning in life for which it is not possible to understand the cause (46). Depression is inextricably linked to mental pain experience: patients may present with aversive, anguished, or uncomfortable emotional states characterized by painful tension and torment, and may become suicidal when they perceive such states as incapable of change (46, 47). However, mental pain can also occur independently from depression. Mental pain may be associated with anxiety disorders, particularly in the perception of invalidism in agoraphobia or a social barrier in social anxiety disorder (46). A simple self-rated clinimetric index, the Mental Pain Questionnaire (MPQ), is available (36, 46). Box 7.4 provides questions that may supplement the

---

Box 7.4 Questions to Address the Identification and Assessment of Mental Pain

---

Mental or psychological pain is an experience that is part of life. It is different from physical pain. We would like to learn about your experience of mental pain:

- Do you feel mental pain that goes beyond what one may experience in life from time to time?
- How does it compare with physical pain?
- Does it hurt all the time or in specific moments? Does it occur every day or less frequently?
- Is there anything that makes it worse or better?
- Do you want to die when you feel it? Do you think that only death will stop it?

---

standard clinical interview. Mental pain is frequently experienced in the setting of tapering and discontinuation of antidepressant drugs, and may be a helpful aid to understanding the clinical state of the patient.

Translating Assessment into a Clinical Decision

When confronted with the different situations described in Chapter 5, the clinician needs a very careful and expanded assessment to be able to reach a decision and to involve the patient in the procedure. An easy objection is that such assessment is too time-consuming and not suited to a busy practice. However, if we compare this procedure with the hidden costs of simply protracting treatments and ignoring the problems, we may realize it is definitely worthwhile. It may also offer otherwise unavailable insights into the patient's symptomatology that prompted the use of antidepressant drugs. Deciding to discontinue the medication could be rather straightforward in situations where there is a lack or loss of clinical effect, or a switch into bipolar disorder. The problem is, however, how and when to discontinue. This is what I will discuss in the following chapters.

References

1. Diagnostic and Statistical Manual of Mental Disorders: Fifth Edition. DSM-5. Washington, DC, American Psychiatric Association, 2013.
2. American Psychiatric Association: Practice Guidelines for the Psychiatric Evaluation of Adults: Third Edition. Arlington, VA, American Psychiatric Publishing, 2017.
3. Fava GA, Rafanelli C, Tomba E: The clinical process in psychiatry: a clinimetric approach. J Clin Psychiatry 2012; 73:177–84.
4. Feinstein AR: The Jones criteria and the challenge of clinimetrics. Circulation 1982; 66:1–5.
5. Feinstein AR: Clinimetrics. New Haven, CT, Yale University Press, 1987.
6. Fava GA, Tomba E, Sonino N: Clinimetrics: the science of clinical measurements. Int J Clin Pract 2012; 66:11–15.
7. Fava GA, Tomba E, Bech P: Clinical pharmacopsychology: conceptual foundations and emerging tasks. Psychother Psychosom 2017; 8:134–40.
8. Moore TJ, Mattison D: Adult utilization of psychiatric drugs and differences by sex, age and race. JAMA Intern Med 2017; 177:274–5.
9. Gnjidic D, Tinetti M, Allore HG: Assessing medication burden and polypharmacy: finding the perfect measure. Expert Rev Clin Pharmacol 2017; 10:345–7.
10. Parker C: Psychiatric effects of drugs for other disorders. Medicine 2016; 44:768–74.
11. Fava GA, Sonino N: Depression associated with medical illness. CNS Drugs 1996; 5:175–89.
12. Patten SB, Barbui C: Drug-induced depression: a systematic review to inform clinical practice. Psychother Psychosom 2004; 73:207–15.
13. Botts S, Ryan M: Depression. In: Tisdale JE, Miller DA (eds). Drug-Induced Diseases. Prevention, Detection and Management. Second Edition. Bethesda, MD, American Society of the Health-System Pharmacists, 2010, pp. 317–32.
14. Qato DM, Ozenberher K, Olfson M: Prevalence of prescription medications with depression as a potential adverse effect among adults in the United States. JAMA 2018; 319:2289–98.
15. Fava GA, Kellner R: Staging: a neglected dimension in psychiatric classification. Acta Psychiatr Scand 1993; 87:225–30.
16. Cosci F, Fava GA: Staging of mental disorders: systematic review. Psychother Psychosom 2013; 82:20–34.
17. Detre TP, Jarecki H. Modern Psychiatric Treatment. Philadelphia, Lippincott, 1971.
18. Fava GA, Cosci F, Guidi J, Rafanelli C: The deceptive manifestations of treatment resistance in depression. Psychother Psychosom 2020; 89:265–73.
19. Cosci F, Chouinard G: Acute and persistent withdrawal syndromes following discontinuation of psychotropic medications. Psychother Psychosom 2020; 89:283–306.
20. Fava GA. Subclinical symptoms in mood disorders: pathophysiological and therapeutic implications. Psychol Med 1999; 29:47–61.
21. Paykel ES: Partial remission, residual symptoms, and relapse in depression. Dialogues Clin Neurosci 2008; 10:431–5.

22. Guidi J, Tomba E, Cosci F, Park SK, Fava GA: The role of staging in planning psychotherapeutic interventions in depression. J Clin Psychiatry 2017; 78:456–63.
23. Diagnostic and Statistical Manual of Mental Disorders: Fourth Edition. DSM-IV. Washington, DC, American Psychiatric Association, 1994.
24. Paykel ES, Tanner J: Life events, depression relapse and maintenance treatment. Psychol Med 1976; 6:481–5.
25. Fava GA, McEwen BS, Guidi J, Gostoli S, Offidani E, Sonino N: Clinical characterization of allostatic overload. Psychoneuroendocrinology 2019; 108:94–101.
26. McEwen BS: Protective and damaging effects of stress mediators. N Engl J Med 1998; 338:171–9.
27. Guidi J, Lucente M, Sonino N, Fava GA: Allostatic load and its impact on health. Psychother Psychosom 2021; 90:11–27.
28. Fava GA, Cosci F, Sonino N: Current psychosomatic practice. Psychother Psychosom 2017; 86:13–30.
29. Fava GA, Guidi J: The pursuit of euthymia. World Psychiatry 2020; 19:40–50.
30. Guidi J, Fava GA: The emerging role of euthymia in psychotherapy research and practice. Clin Psychol Rev 2020; 82:101941.
31. Feinstein AR: The pre-therapeutic classification of comorbidity in chronic disease. J Chronic Dis 1970; 23:455–68.
32. deGroot V, Beckerman H, Lankhorst GJ, Bouter LM: How to measure comorbidity: a critical review of available methods. J Clin Epidemiol 2003; 56:221–9.
33. Emmelkamp PMG, Bouman TK, Scholing A: Anxiety Disorders. Chichester, Wiley, 1993.
34. Fava GA, Sonino N, Wise TN (eds): The Psychosomatic Assessment. Basel, Karger, 2012.
35. Fava M: Diagnosis and definition of treatment-resistant depression. Biol Psychiatry 2003; 53:649–59.
36. Fava GA: Well-Being Therapy. Treatment Manual and Clinical Applications. Basel, Karger, 2016.
37. Chouinard G, Chouinard VA: New classification of selective serotonin reuptake inhibitor withdrawal. Psychother Psychosom 2015; 84:63–71.
38. Rosenbaum JF, Fava M, Hoog SL, Ascroft C, Krebs WB: Selective serotonin reuptake inhibitor discontinuation syndrome: a randomized clinical trial. Biol Psychiatry 1998; 44:77–87.
39. Cosci F, Chouinard G, Chouinard V-A, Fava GA: The Diagnostic Clinical Interview for Drug Withdrawal 1(DID-W1)—new symptoms of selective serotonin reuptake inhibitors (SSRI) or serotonin noradrenaline reuptake inhibitors (SNRI): inter-rater reliability. Riv Psichiat 2018; 53:95–9.
40. Papp A, Onton JA: Brain zaps: an underappreciated symptom of antidepressant discontinuation. Prim Care Companion CNS Disord 2018; 20:18m2311.
41. Baldessarini RJ, Tondo L: Effects of treatment discontinuation in clinical psychopharmacology. Psychother Psychosom 2019; 88:65–70.
42. Cohen D, Recalt AM: Discontinuing psychotropic drugs from participants in randomized controlled trials. Psychother Psychosom 2019; 88:96–104.
43. Recalt AM, Cohen S: Withdrawal confounding in randomized controlled trials of antipsychotic, antidepressant, and stimulant drugs, 2000–2017. Psychother Psychosom 2019; 88:105–13.

44. Guidi J, Fava GA, Bech P, Paykel E: The Clinical Interview for Depression. Psychother Psychosom 2011; 80:10–27.

45. Carrozzino D, Patierno C, Fava GA, Guidi J: The Hamilton Rating Scales for Depression. Psychother Psychosom 2020; 89:133–50.

46. Fava GA, Tomba E, Brakemeier EL, Carrozzino D, Cosci F, Eory A, Leonardi T, Schamong I, Guidi J: Mental pain as a transdiagnostic patient-reported outcome measure. Psychother Psychosom 2019; 88:341–9.

47. Alacreu-Crespo A, Cazals A, Courtet P, Olié E: Brief assessment of psychological pain to predict suicidal events at one year in depressed patients. Psychother Psychosom 2020; 89:320–3.

8

Pharmacological Strategies and Options

Up to a few years ago, there was consensus in the literature (1–4), as summarized by Wilson and Lader (5), that antidepressant medications should be tapered as slowly as possible, over at least 4 weeks or longer, and that the same antidepressant should be reinstated if discontinuation symptoms occurred. Another suggested procedure was to switch to fluoxetine, which is less likely than other SSRIs to induce discontinuation problems (6). Such recommendations were soon incorporated in mainstream psychiatry, because of their reassuring connotation in terms of pharmaceutical interests (withdrawal syndromes were disguised as harmless discontinuation problems). However, they were not based on controlled studies and mainly reflected the interpretations and clinical experiences of the authors. Also today, proper RCTs on how to manage the discontinuation of antidepressant drugs are missing.

What I describe in this and the following chapters thus reflects my clinical experience, which is likely to be heavily biased in relation to my type of practice and my interpretative schemas, such as the oppositional model of tolerance. I will try to outline the dilemmas and potential solutions that the clinician encounters when confronted with the various situations, referring to both the literature that is available on various aspects of antidepressant medications and my clinical and conceptual appraisal of the problem. It is wishful thinking to believe that there is a single protocol, as endorsed in clinical guidelines, that can be applied to all patients for whom antidepressant drugs are discontinued. In any event, the fear of opening Pandora's box, by researchers in the field, has been so great that even the guidelines fail to provide any specific direction.

The American Psychiatric Association guidelines (7) are a good example of the tendency to minimize the frequency and seriousness of withdrawal reactions and of the vagueness of the management indications:

Discontinuation-emergent symptoms include both flu-like experiences such as nausea, headache, light-headedness, chills, and body aches, and neurological symptoms such as paresthesias, insomnia, and "electric shock-like" phenomena. These symptoms typically resolve without specific treatment over 1–2 weeks. However, some patients do experience more protracted discontinuation syndromes, particularly those treated with paroxetine, and may require a slower downward titration regimen. (7, p. 37)

My current interpretation and orientation as to the management of withdrawal reactions also reflect some changes in my clinical appraisal that have occurred over the years. When, in the nineties, I started being confronted with withdrawal reactions from antidepressant medications, I followed what appeared then to be the most reasonable approach. First, I thought it was necessary to reduce newer-generation antidepressants at a slower pace than TCAs (whose smallest decrement was, for instance, 25 mg of imipramine every other week). I discovered that, in some patients, tapering and discontinuing SSRIs and SNRIs was relatively easy, while in other patients it aroused withdrawal symptoms and mental pain, no matter how slowly I tried, with new withdrawal symptoms occurring also during tapering. Indeed, the idea that you could avoid withdrawal reactions simply by discontinuing medications slowly—which is why antidepressants were supposedly different from other psychotropic drugs (1–5)—was not supported either by my experience or by the published literature (8, 9). I was unable to identify valid predictors of the occurrence of withdrawal syndromes, except when paroxetine and venlaxine were involved, and this was also confirmed by our analyses of the literature (8, 9). I tried to see whether stopping for some time (e.g., a month) at a specific dosage during tapering (e.g., 10 mg of paroxetine/day) could help. It did not. Once the antidepressant medication was discontinued and the withdrawal syndrome did not subside within a few weeks, I started the same antidepressant again, when requested by the patient. It seldom worked, and it was not surprising to me because of the links with another form of behavioral toxicity—resistance (see Chapter 3). Neither did the switch to fluoxetine seem to work.

Sharing views and experiences with colleagues in the academic field might be another source of help, but I was frustrated by the fact that, today, so few researchers actually assess, treat, and follow up patients outside of clinical studies. Fortunately, Guy Chouinard provided some important insights. He had suggested the potential use of anticonvulsants, particularly gabapentin and lamotrigine, to decrease the intensity of withdrawal (10). However, because the majority of my patients who were struggling to discontinue antidepressants had anxiety disorders, I became more interested in clonazepam, a BZ with specific anticonvulsant properties, which Chouinard himself had introduced into clinical use for panic disorder and bipolar illness (11). I thought that its anti-anxiety and mood-modulating properties could be very suitable for decreasing withdrawal symptomatology. Further, I was aware of its effectiveness as cotherapy with SSRIs in conditions such as panic disorder (12), and of the preclinical evidence linking it with serotonergic activity (13, 14). I was also impressed by the results of clonazepam for managing the paradoxical manifestations of depression in patients with anxiety disorders treated with SSRIs (15). Finally, I had successfully used clonazepam as a prophylactic therapy in depressed patients who underwent sequential treatment and had a relapse (16). First, I used clonazepam only if new withdrawal symptoms appeared ("wait and see" approach). Then, I started using it with all patients with newer-generation antidepressants, regardless of the appearance of withdrawal symptomatology. I became convinced that one needs a medication other than an antidepressant in the discontinuation process.

Working in a multidisciplinary team, I could appreciate the importance of associating specific psychotherapeutic approaches with the management of discontinuation of antidepressant drugs. In particular, with Carlotta Belaise, we developed modules and plans of psychotherapy that could enhance pharmacological strategies (17, 18). I also realized the importance of having a consultant internist, Nicoletta Sonino, with a deep knowledge of the medical problems that may occur in psychiatric settings.

I will first describe the sequential structure of these modules, and then the specific pharmacological problems that may ensue with discontinuing antidepressant drugs.

Structure and Staging of the Interventions

The information obtained using the assessment described in the previous chapter allows any decision to be set in the specific context of the individual patient.

First, there may be all the indications for attempting a discontinuation of antidepressant medications, but the presence of the following circumstances may suggest its postponement to a later point in time:

1. **Allostatic overload** The condition is often precipitated by the addition of recent stressful life circumstances to an ongoing situation of chronic stress (19). In view of the close relationship between life events and relapse in depression (20), it is not the right time to add the potential burden of withdrawal symptoms to a situation of allostatic overload. Yet, I observed that many patients request that medication is stopped just when they are most stressed.

2. **Unstable medical conditions** An important prerequisite before discontinuation is that the patient is medically stable. Bainum et al. (21) reported on the severe consequences of the abrupt discontinuation of antidepressants (e.g., delirium, agitation, irritability) in patients who are critically ill. Further, and often, if the patient taking antidepressant drugs is hospitalized for events such as minor elective surgery, these medications are forgotten or discontinued, which may cause serious problems. On the other hand, there are medical complications, such as cardiac problems or gastrointestinal bleeding, which may dictate a rapid discontinuation of the antidepressant medications that may be related to them (22), as indicated in Box 5.1 (see p. 48).

3. **Mood instability** Similar considerations apply to the presence of mood instability and high reactivity to environmental stimuli despite antidepressant therapy. Even for patients with alleged unipolar depression (particularly if a history of behavioral toxicity is present), the time may not be favorable. In patients with bipolar disorder, antidepressant medications should never be tapered without the concomitant use of mood stabilizers. Even though, in principle, antidepressants are likely to affect unfavorably the course of bipolar illness and their removal may thus be viewed as positive, the

instability they may cause in terms of withdrawal reactions may add to subclinical fluctuations that already occur in the disorder (23).

Clinical judgment should thus evaluate the pros and cons of each clinical situation, as well as the basic protocol that we developed for discontinuing antidepressant medications (17) (Figure 8.1).

For instance, antidepressant discontinuation may take place in stage 1 if there are indications for its rapid execution, as I am going to describe in the next section. In the case of patients with anxiety disorders, obsessive-compulsive disorder, and post-traumatic stress disorder—who were never offered or benefited from cognitive-behavioral methods or other evidence-based psychotherapies and are on maintenance antidepressant treatment—the likelihood of early relapse is so high at 1 year (24) that a different modulation may be advised (Figure 8.2). There is thus the need of addressing symptoms such as phobias and obsessions with psychotherapeutic methods before attempting a discontinuation of antidepressant drugs.

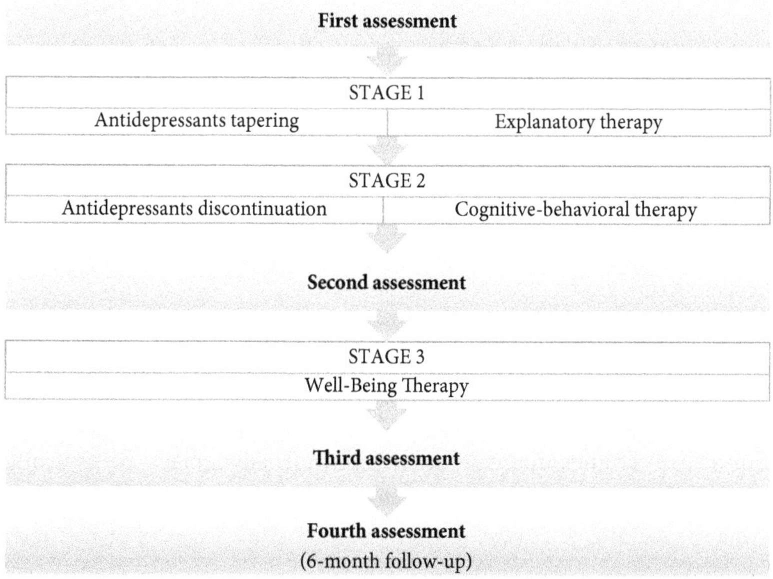

First assessment

STAGE 1	
Antidepressants tapering	Explanatory therapy

STAGE 2	
Antidepressants discontinuation	Cognitive-behavioral therapy

Second assessment

STAGE 3
Well-Being Therapy

Third assessment

Fourth assessment
(6-month follow-up)

Figure 8.1 Staging of Pharmacological and Psychotherapeutic Interventions for Discontinuation of Antidepressants

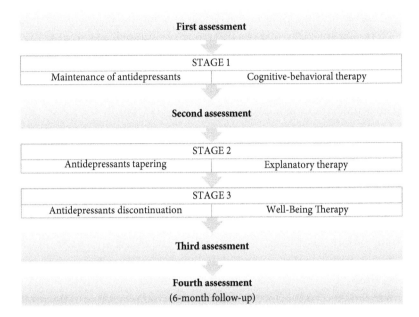

First assessment

STAGE 1	
Maintenance of antidepressants	Cognitive-behavioral therapy

Second assessment

STAGE 2	
Antidepressants tapering	Explanatory therapy

STAGE 3	
Antidepressants discontinuation	Well-Being Therapy

Third assessment

Fourth assessment
(6-month follow-up)

Figure 8.2 Alternative Staging of Pharmacological and Psychotherapeutic Interventions for Discontinuation of Antidepressants

In addition to the initial evaluation, full assessments are necessary after antidepressant discontinuation and completion of CBT (Figure 8.1) or completion of WBT and antidepressant discontinuation (Figure 8.2). With both modalities, another full examination 6 months after antidepressant discontinuation is essential to evaluate the potential occurrence of persistent postwithdrawal disorder and relapse.

Methods of Discontinuation and Pharmacological Approaches

Controlled studies indicate no significant advantages of tapering compared to abrupt discontinuation as to onset of withdrawal symptoms (8, 9, 25–27). However, there is an entire spectrum of methods for tapering antidepressant medications, which can range from a few weeks to several months, in relation to the initial dosage, the amount of each decrease, and the intervals between steps. For instance, if we have a patient who takes 20 mg of citalopram/day, we may decide to split a tablet and discontinue citalopram after 2 weeks. Or we may decide, with the use of liquid formulation, to perform smaller steps with longer intervals. Online tapering information suggests a 10% reduction per month (28). Scholten et al. (29) indicated time intervals of at least 4 weeks (for fluoxetine, 3 months) and that when withdrawal symptoms have not disappeared by that time, the interval should be extended. A very slow strategy has recently been suggested by Horowitz and Taylor (30). Reviewing positron emission tomography imaging data, they suggested that SSRIs should be taken hyperbolically, initially relatively quickly, but then progressively more slowly, to very small doses (lower than minimum therapeutic doses), in a process that may take months. These very small decrements may be achieved with liquid formulations of antidepressants or with personal tapering strips (31). As a result, we can have relatively rapid tapering based on availability of tablets, regardless of the persistence of withdrawal symptoms before the next step, extending over weeks; or we can have slow and ultra-slow tapering extending over months or years. Currently, there is no evidence based on RCTs to suggest that very slow methods yield better results than faster modalities.

Regardless of the method that is chosen, the availability for frequent contacts (one for each step) appears to be essential. Tapering with frequent contacts appears to be a reasonable general clinical strategy. Even though it may not produce advantages as to the likelihood of withdrawal symptoms (and certainly not of postwithdrawal phenomena), it allows close monitoring of the clinical situation. Yet, there may be situations where abrupt interruption may be the most viable choice and other situations where the rate of tapering is dictated by the clinical circumstance (e.g., a pregnant woman who wants to discontinue the antidepressant as soon as possible). There are advantages and disadvantages with each choice. Slower methods may reduce the severity of withdrawal reactions and be more acceptable to the patient (even though this remains to be demonstrated); however, such methods extend the exposure to antidepressant drugs and potentially increase the manifestations of behavioral toxicity (32).

Once again, the initial decision should be based on clinical judgment and shared with the patient; it can be modified in the course of treatment.

Among the factors to be taken into consideration, the following have particular importance:

1. **Previous experiences with discontinuation of antidepressant drugs** If the patient has attempted to stop antidepressant medications in the past, then the outcome (e.g., severe withdrawal, failure to discontinue) and how these events were perceived and interpreted by the patient should be evaluated. The staging, in terms of behavioral toxicity (see Box 7.2, p. 69), may indicate the level of risk.

2. **Type and duration of current treatment with an antidepressant drug** Patients on paroxetine, venlafaxine, and des-venlafaxine are at high risk of developing withdrawal syndromes compared to other medications in the same class or in other classes. Further, it is a different thing entirely to attempt discontinuation in a patient who has been taking an antidepressant (e.g., paroxetine) for 10–20 years (as I happen to see) as compared to a patient who has been taking the same antidepressant for a few weeks or months. Even though a clear relationship between duration of treatment and dependence with antidepressants has not been established (8, 9), the clinician may be inclined to discontinue a relatively brief treatment as soon as possible, particularly in cases where it was not warranted from the very beginning.

3. **Medical and psychiatric side effects** These include both the presence of conditions requiring urgent medical attention (see Box 5.1, p. 48) and the occurrence of paradoxical effects and/or a switch into bipolar disorder, which call for rapid discontinuation of the antidepressant medications.

4. **Patient's preference** This is a very important factor (shared decision-making) that requires appropriate information (see Chapter 9) and the possibility to change opinion. For instance, a patient on paroxetine opted for slow tapering, but when the withdrawal symptoms ensued he expressed the following wish: "It is hell, and I now realize it is like a poison; please help me get it out of my body as soon as possible, no matter how much I have to suffer." Some patients may thus express the wish to discontinue treatment abruptly in order to

curtail the period in which withdrawal symptoms are experienced during tapering (33).

Abrupt or two-step rapid tapering may be considered when switching from one antidepressant therapy to another due to lack or loss of efficacy. The value of tapering one antidepressant and introducing the other during tapering or after discontinuation has not been established. Keks et al. (34) outlined various techniques that range from a conservative switch (the first antidepressant is gradually reduced and stopped, followed by a washout period after which the new antidepressant is started) to a direct switch (the first antidepressant is stopped; the other is started the next day) via a cross-taper switch (the new antidepressant is introduced as the first is reduced). It is important to remember, however, that these strategies do not apply to MAO inhibitors, for which specific recommendations should be followed (34). In my clinical experience, abrupt switching may be preferable—warning the patient about the intermediate phase when withdrawal symptoms of the first drug may occur and the benefits of the new one may not have appeared yet. As I discuss in Chapter 13, caution is needed in changing antidepressants in treatment-resistant depression, owing to the risk of inducing a cascade iatrogenesis (35).

As I previously mentioned and described in some case illustrations, I tend to use rapid tapering (splitting the tablets of an antidepressant or using lower dosages as in the case of venlafaxine)—with intervals of 2 weeks, which may be extended slightly in relation to environmental situations (allostatic load)—in combination with clonazepam. I add clonazepam to the antidepressant I want to discontinue and, after 2 weeks of stabilization, I start tapering. I start clonazepam at very low doses (0.25 mg twice/day). The BZ may be increased when withdrawal symptomatology worsens (up to 4 mg/day): it appears to decrease, though not eliminate, the intensity of symptoms. As withdrawal symptomatology may persist for months and build up into postwithdrawal disorders, clonazepam treatment may also need to be protracted. Similar considerations apply to the case of anxiety disorders that cannot be treated with psychotherapy. The choice of clonazepam is based on its anti-anxiety properties, paucity of side effects, facility to titrate, paucity of significant interactions, mood-modulating effects, value in conjunction with or after antidepressants, and low likelihood for dependence compared to other BZs (11, 36, 37). Needless to say, we would need a double-blind placebo-controlled trial to test this approach and these clinical impressions. An important objection to introducing clonazepam may be that we simply change from one type of dependence to another (38). This may be true, but the clinical manifestations in discontinuing antidepressant medications appear to be much worse than with BZs (38). In line with the published literature (39), I did not encounter significant problems in tapering and discontinuing clonazepam at some time after the discontinuation of the antidepressant drug.

Reintroducing the antidepressant that was first used or switching from one antidepressant to another (such as fluoxetine) to suppress clinical manifestations of withdrawal (1–5) are both highly questionable suggestions that are no longer tenable. A rational use of drugs depends on the balance of potential benefits and adverse effects as applied to the individual patient. It is one thing to reinstate an antidepressant if relapse has occurred; it is quite another thing to do it if withdrawal has ensued. In the latter case, we should be aware that we are simply postponing, and most likely aggravating, the problem (17). Tolerance may occur as a reaction to particular effects of a drug that may be shared by medications of the same class. In our model of tolerance (32), the same opponent processes (most likely involving 5-HT1A autoreceptors) may be activated by different antidepressants. As a result, if we administer an antidepressant medication, regardless of whether it is the same or a different one, we may worsen the state of behavioral toxicity which is associated with withdrawal phenomena, as well as other manifestations of oppositional tolerance (32). I thus avoid using antidepressant drugs in case of withdrawal symptoms, even though I may be forced to use antidepressant therapy, for the shortest possible time, for mood fluctuations in persistent postwithdrawal disorders which reach the intensity threshold of a major depressive disorder and do not respond to clonazepam treatment and psychotherapeutic interventions. In this case, as suggested by Fux et al. (15), I use a TCA at low doses (e.g., clomipramine 50 mg/day). Once again, the appropriateness of this practice should be verified by a RCT.

Finally, a specific problem involves the occurrence of hypomania or mania in conjunction with new withdrawal symptomatology (40, 41).

The syndrome may be self-limiting (although seldom in my experience). Clonazepam, despite its antimanic properties, is unlikely to control it, and hypomania/mania may require specific mood-stabilizing treatment as in the case of Robert in Chapter 3.

Interactions with Other Medications

A clinical issue that has attracted little attention concerns the interactions between antidepressant drugs, particularly SSRIs and SNRIs, with a number of other medical drugs. Tapering and discontinuing antidepressants may require readjustment of medical therapies, which once again emphasizes the need for medical consultation (see Chapter 6). In particular, with first-generation antidepressants, caution is needed with oral anticoagulants (warfarin, dicumarol), antihypertensive agents, levodopa, and anticholinergic agents (42). With newer-generation antidepressants (particularly with SSRIs and SNRIs), one should keep in mind that they are generally extensively metabolized in the liver by cytochrome P450 and may thus be the target of metabolically-based drug interactions (43). Again, caution is needed, especially with oral anticoagulants, antihypertensive agents, antiarrhythmic agents, anticonvulsants, antifungal agents, corticosteroids, immunosuppressants, protein pump inhibitors, statins, and tamoxifen (44, 45). There might be major differences within the broad class of newer-generation antidepressants (e.g., between mirtazapine and SSRIs), and the clinician is urged to check manuals (44–48) and online resources (which may be particularly important for newly-released compounds). It is simply astonishing how these crucial clinical issues are ignored in guidelines and reviews that are supposed to inform clinical practice.

A further issue in discontinuing antidepressants has to do with the frequent practice of polypharmacy in medicine (49) and psychiatry (50). If we have a patient who is taking paroxetine, quetiapine, and triazolam, how are we going to proceed? All three drugs are very likely to cause dependence and withdrawal symptoms. While it appears to be obvious that they cannot all be discontinued at the same time, there are unanswered clinical questions: Which drug should we stop first? What is the cross-tolerance of the drugs (i.e., how do they affect each other in terms of withdrawal symptomatology)? Polypharmacy is simply not addressed by the literature on antidepressant discontinuation, and yet it is a frequently encountered clinical reality. Assessing the medication burden and polypharmacy (49) is thus another important factor in selecting discontinuation strategies. Macroanalysis can incorporate the iatrogenic comorbidity potentially entailed by psychotropic drugs and be a helpful ground for placing priority on specific choices based on clinical reasoning.

Monitoring and Managing the Clinical Course After Discontinuation

The repeated psychiatric assessments that are described in Figures 8.1 and 8.2 offer the opportunity to monitor the clinical course after discontinuing antidepressant medications: specifically, whether new withdrawal symptoms occur (see Box 2.1, p. 13) and reach the threshold of a syndrome (see Box 2.2, p. 16); whether they subside in the course of time or build up into a persistent postwithdrawal disorder (see Box 2.3, p. 17); whether there is return of the original symptoms, also at a greater intensity; and, finally, the potential appearance of new symptoms/disorders that were not present before. This latter occurrence may be particularly troublesome and justifies a careful examination 6 months after discontinuation of antidepressant medications. Longitudinal studies exploring the occurrence, clinical features, and neurobiological correlates of persistent postwithdrawal disorders are needed. In a recent longitudinal epidemiological investigation (51), mood disorders were found to be associated with an increased risk of developing other mental disorders. A possibility that needs to be explored, and was not entertained by the authors, is that antidepressant treatment, more than depression itself, might have caused persistent postwithdrawal disorders and be, at least in part, responsible for the increased comorbidity. Such studies are now feasible since diagnostic criteria are available (10, 38).

The psychotherapeutic modules that I am going to describe in the following chapters have the aim of addressing symptoms that would otherwise require drug treatment and of preventing the progression of new withdrawal symptoms to persistent postwithdrawal disorder (once again, to be verified by RCTs). In some cases, however, psychotherapeutic treatment, no matter how skillful, may be unable to counteract anxious and depressive symptoms. Clonazepam may be similarly ineffective, and the reintroduction of the original or similar antidepressant medication runs counter to any clinical sense. One may need to introduce new psychotropic medications such as antiepilepetic drugs, as suggested by Chouinard and Chouinard (10), or low doses of a TCA for a brief period of time. When the persistent postwithdrawal disorder takes the form of mood swings, which may approach the criteria for cyclothymic disorder, the use of lithium may be warranted. Repeated medical assessments by the consulting internist may also be necessary in case of comorbid medical conditions and treatments.

Not Just a Medication Check

Biological reductionism, neglect of individual responses to treatment, massive pharmaceutical propaganda, and a lack of consideration of multiple therapeutic ingredients and incremental care have deeply affected psychiatric practice (52). This approach has created a split between pharmacological and psychological treatments. The role of psychiatrists within public mental health clinics has been hampered by a perceived restriction of this to prescribing and signing forms, limiting opportunities to engage in the kind of integrated care that attracted many physicians to this specialty (52). Therapeutic ingredients of a psychological nature do not exclusively take the route of formal psychotherapy with an established number of sessions, generally nowadays performed by psychologists or other qualified workers in the mental health field. They may take the form of psychotherapeutic management, i.e., the application of psychological understanding to the management and rehabilitation of the individual patient (53). Such an approach includes establishing a therapeutic relationship, helping the patient to identify and deal with current life problems, providing lifestyle suggestions, and working with his/her family and significant others (53, 54). It may also include selecting some simple and specific ingredients extracted from psychotherapeutic protocols. Antidepressant drugs are therapeutic tools of modest efficacy in a specific setting characterized by the clinician's full availability to answering patient's questions, the patient's opportunity to ventilate thoughts and feelings, the development of a patient–doctor interaction, and the perception of competent care (54–57). When these nonspecific therapeutic ingredients are missing, drugs are unlikely to be superior to placebo (58).

The physician's approach to discontinuing antidepressant medications cannot be exempt from psychotherapeutic management. As with the sequential model, the physician may decide to carry out, himself/herself, the psychotherapeutic modules included in our treatment strategy (see Chapters 9–11) or, more realistically, delegate these modules to the clinical psychologists in the treatment team (see Chapter 6). However, psychotherapeutic management—with particular reference to the first module described in the next chapter—should never be omitted.

References

1. Lojoyeux M, Ades J: Antidepressant discontinuation. J Clin Psychiatry 1997; 58 (suppl. 7):11–16.
2. Haddad PM: Antidepressant discontinuation syndromes. Drug Safety 2001; 24:183–97.
3. Schatzberg AF, Blier P, Delgado PL, Fava M, Haddad PM, Shelton RC: Antidepressant discontinuation syndrome. J Clin Psychiatry 2006; 67 (suppl. 4):27–30.
4. Warner CH, Bobo W, Warner C, Reid S, Rachal J: Antidepressant discontinuation syndrome. Am Fam Physician 2006; 74:449–56.
5. Wilson E, Lader M: A review of the management of antidepressant discontinuation symptoms. Ther Adv Psychopharmacol 2015; 5:357–8.
6. Rosenbaum JF, Fava M, Hoog SL, Ascroft C, Krebs WB: Selective serotonin reuptake inhibitor discontinuation syndrome: a randomized clinical trial. Biol Psychiatry 1998; 44:77–87.
7. American Psychiatric Association: Practice guideline for the treatment of patients with major depressive disorder. Third edition. Am J Psychiatry 2010;167 (Suppl.):1–118.
8. Fava GA, Gatti A, Belaise C, Guidi J, Offidani E: Withdrawal symptoms after selective serotonin reuptake inhibitor discontinuation: a systematic review. Psychother Psychosom 2015; 84:72–81.
9. Fava GA, Benasi G, Lucente M, Offidani E, Cosci F, Guidi J: Withdrawal symptoms after serotonin-noradrenaline reuptake inhibitor discontinuation. Psychother Psychosom 2018; 87:195–203.
10. Chouinard G, Chouinard VA: New classification of selective serotonin reuptake inhibitor withdrawal. Psychother Psychosom 2015; 84:63–71.

11. Chouinard G: Issues in the clinical use of benzodiazepines: potency, withdrawal and rebound. J Clin Psychiatry 2004; 65 (Suppl. 5):7–12.

12. Goddard AW, Brouette T, Almai A, Jett P, Woods S, Charney D: Early coadministration of clonazepam with sertraline for panic disorder. Arch Gen Psychiatry 2001; 58:681–6.

13. Pratt J, Jenner P, Reynolds EH, Marsden CD: Clonazepam induces decreased serotonin activity in the mouse barin. Neuropharmacology 1979; 18:791–9.

14. Lima l, Trejo E, Urbina M: Serotonin turnover rate, ^{3}H paroxetine binding sites, and -5-HT1a receptors in the hippocampus of rats subcronically treated with clonazepam. Neuropharmacology 1995; 34:1327–33.

15. Fux M, Taub M, Zohar J: Emergence of depressive symptoms during treatment for panic disorder with specific 5-hydroxytryptophan reuptake inhibitors. Acta Psychiatr Scand 1993; 88:235–7.

16. Fava GA, Ruini C, Rafanelli C, Finos L, Conti S, Grandi S: Six-year outcome of cognitive behavior therapy for prevention of recurrent depression. Am J Psychiatry 2004; 161:1872–6.

17. Fava GA, Belaise C: Discontinuing antidepressants drugs: lesson from a failed trial and extensive clinical experience. Psychother Psychosom 2018; 87:257–67.

18. Belaise C, Gatti A, Chouinard VA, Chouinard G: Persistent postwithdrawal disorders induced by paroxetine, a selective serotonin reuptake inhibitor, and treated with specific cognitive behavioral therapy. Psychother Psychosom 2014; 83:247–8.

19. Fava GA, McEwen BS, Guidi J, Gostoli S, Offidani E, Sonino N: Clinical characterization of allostatic overload. Psychoneuroendocrinology 2019; 108:94–101.

20. Paykel ES, Tanner J: Life events, depression relapse and maintenance treatment. Psychol Med 1976; 6:481–5.

21. Bainum TB, Fike DS, Mechelay D, Haase K: Effect of abrupt discontinuation of antidepressants in critically ill hospitalized patients. Pharmacotherapy 2017; 37:1231–40.

22. Carvalho AF, Sharma MS, Brunoni AR, Vieta E, Fava GA: The safety, tolerability and risks associated with the use of newer generation antidepressant drugs. Psychother Psychosom 2016; 85:270–88.

23. Fava GA, Cosci F, Offidani J, Guidi J: Behavioral toxicity revisited. J Clin Psychopharmacol 2016; 36:550–3.

24. Batelaan NM, Bosman RC, Muntingh A, Scholten WD, Huijbregts KM, van Balkom AJLM: Risk of relapse after antidepressant discontinuation in anxiety disorders, obsessive-compulsive disorder, and post-traumatic stress disorder. BMJ 2017; 358:j3927.

25. Tint A, Haddad PM, Anderson IM: The effect of rate of antidepressant tapering on the incidence of discontinuation symptoms: a randomised study. J Psychopharmacol 2008; 22:330–2.

26. Gallagher J, Strzinek RA, Cheng RJ, Ausmanas MK, Astl, D, Seljan P: The effect of dose titration and dose tapering on the tolerability of desvenlafaxine in women with vasomotor symptoms associated with menopause. J Women's Health 2012; 21:188–98.

27. Khan A, Musgnung J, Ramey T, Messig M, Buckley G, Ninan P: Abrupt discontinuation compared with a 1-week taper regimen in depressed outpatients

treated for 24 weeks with desvenlafaxine 50 mg/d. J Clin Psychopharmacol 2014; 34:365–8.

28. Hengartner MP, Schulthess L, Sorensen A, Framer A: Protracted withdrawal syndrome after stopping antidepressants. Ther Adv Psychopharmacology 2020 Dec 24; 10:2045125320980573.

29. Scholten W, Batelaan N, van Balkom A: Barriers to discontinuing antidepressants in patients with depressive and anxiety disorders. Ther Adv Psychopharmacology 2020 Jun 10; 10:2045125320933404.

30. Horowitz MA, Taylor D: Tapering of SSRI treatment to mitigate withdrawal symptoms. Lancet Psychiatry 2019; 6:538–46.

31. Groot PC, van Os J: How user knowledge of psychotropic drug withdrawal resulted in the development of person-specific tapering medication. Ther Adv Psychopharmacology 2020 Jul 10; 10:2045125320932452.

32. Fava GA: May antidepressant drugs worsen the conditions they are supposed to treat? The clinical foundations of the oppositional model of tolerance. Ther Adv Psychopharmacol 2020; Nov 2; 10:2045125320970325.

33. Haddad PM: Antidepressant discontinuation syndromes. Drug Safety 2001; 24:183–97.

34. Keks N, Hope J, Keogh S: Switching and stopping antidepressants. Aust Prescr 2016; 39:76–83.

35. Fava GA, Cosci F, Guidi J, Rafanelli C: The deceptive manifestations of treatment resistance in depression. Psychother Psychosom 2020; 89:265–73.

36. Pollack MH, Van Ameringen M, Simon N, Worthinton JW, Hoge EA, Keshaviah A, Stein MB: A double-blind randomized controlled trial of augmentation and switch strategies for refractory social anxiety disorder. Am J Psychiatry 2014; 171:44–53.

37. Cloos JM, Bocquet V, Rolland-Portal I, Koch P, Chouinard G: Hypnotics and triazolobenzodiazepines—best predictors of high-dose benzodiazepine use. Psychother Psychosom 2015; 84:273–83.

38. Cosci F, Chouinard G: Acute and persistent withdrawal syndromes following discontinuation of psychotropic medications. Psychother Psychosom 2020; 89:283–306.

39. Nardi AE, Freire RC, Valenca AM, Amrein R, de Cerqueira CR, Lopes FL, Nascimento I, Mezzaslama MA, Veras AB, Sardinha A, de Carvalho MR, da Costa RT, Levitan MN, de Melo-Neto VL, Soares-Filho GL, Versiani M: Tapering clonazepam in patients with panic disorder after at least 3 years of treatment. J Clin Psychopharmacol 2010; 30:290–3.

40. Andrade C: Antidepressant-withdrawal mania. J Clin Psychiatry 2004; 65:987–93.

41. Tomba E, Guidi J, Fava GA: What psychologists need to know about psychotropic medications. Clin Psychol Psychother 2018; 25:181–7.

42. Fava GA, Sonino N: Depression associated with medical illness. CNS Drugs 1996; 5:175–89.

43. Spina E, Trifirò G, Caraci F: Clinically significant drug interactions with newer antidepressants. CNS Drugs 2012; 26:39–67.

44. Procyshyn RM, Bezchlibnyk-Butler KZ, Jeffries JJ (eds): Clinical Handbook of Psychotropic Drugs. 23rd Edition. Boston, Hogrefe, 2019.

45. Ciraulo DA, Shader RI, Greenblatt DJ, Creelman W (eds): Drug Interactions in Psychiatry. Third Edition. Baltimore, Williams and Wilkins, 2005.
46. Dubovsky SL: Clinical Guide to Psychotropic Drugs. New York, Norton, 2005.
47. Baldessarini RJ: Chemotherapy in Psychiatry. Pharmacologic Basis of Treatments for Major Mental Illness. Third Edition. New York, Springer, 2013.
48. Ghaemi SN: Clinical Psychopharmacology. Principles and Practice. New York, Oxford University Press, 2019.
49. Gnjidic D, Tinetti M, Allore HG: Assessing medication burden and polypharmacy: finding the perfect measure. Exp Rev Clin Pharmacol 2017; 10:345–7.
50. Ghaemi SN (ed): Polypharmacy in Psychiatry. New York, Dekker, 2002.
51. Plana Ripoli O, Pedersen CB, Holtz Y, Benros ME, Dalsgaard S, de Jonge P, Fan CC, Degenhardt L, Ganna A, Greve AN, Gunn J, Iburg KM, Kessing LV, Lee BK, Lim CCW, Mors O, Nordentoft M, Prior A, Roest AM, Saha S, Schork A, Scott JG, Scott KM, Stedman T, Sørensen HJ, Werge T, Whiteford HA, Laursen TM, Agerbo E, Kessler RC, Mortensen PB, McGrath JJ: Exploring comorbidity within mental disorders among a Danish national population. JAMA Psychiatry 2019; 76:259–70.
52. Fava GA, Park SK, Dubovsky SL: The mental health clinic: a new model. World Psychiatry 2008; 7:177–81.
53. Simpson GM, May PRA: Schizophrenic disorders. In: Greist JH, Jefferson JW, Spitzer RL (eds). Treatment of Mental Disorders. New York, Oxford University Press, 1982, pp. 143–83.
54. Fava GA: Modern psychiatric treatment. Psychother Psychosom 2013; 82:1–7.
55. Gliedman CH, Nash EH, Huber SD, Stone AR, Frank JD: Reduction of symptoms by pharmacologically inert substances and by short-term psychotherapy. AMA Arch Neurol Psychiatry 1958; 79:345–51.
56. Downing RW, Rickels K: Nonspecific factors and their interaction with psychological treatment in pharmacotherapy. In: Lipton MA, Di Mascio A, Killam KF (eds). Psychopharmacology: A Generation of Progress. New York, Raven Press, 1978, pp. 1419–27.
57. Fava GA, Guidi J, Rafanelli C, Rickels K: The clinical inadequacy of the placebo model and the development of an alternative conceptual framework. Psychother Psychosom 2017; 86:332–340.
58. Uhlenhuth EN, Rickels K, Fisher S, Park LC, Lipman RS, Mock J: Drug, doctor's verbal attitude and clinic setting in the symptomatic response to pharmacotherapy. Psychopharmacologia 1966; 9:392–418.

9

First Psychotherapeutic Module

Explanatory Therapy

Illness behavior refers to the "varying ways individuals respond to bodily indications, how they monitor internal states, define and interpret symptoms, make attributions, take remedial actions and utilize various sources of informal and formal care" (1). Illness behavior, in its experiential, cognitive, and behavioral aspects, is an important factor in modulating the individual response to the emergence and persistence of new withdrawal symptoms. What the patient perceives represents the experiential aspect; the way he/she interprets such perceptions constitutes the cognitive aspect; and the role of the patient in collaborating with the treatment plan (self-therapy) constitutes the behavioral aspect. The role of illness behavior has been emphasized in medical settings, with particular reference to functional medical disorders (2, 3). There has been less interest in exploring its modulatory effect as to psychiatric symptomatology (4) and psychopharmacology (5). In studying the effects of personality on withdrawal severity and taper outcome in BZ-dependent patients, it has been observed that there are patients who seem to be particularly sensitive to internal cues and are therefore extremely fearful of completing the BZ taper (6). Personality may certainly have a role; however, a certain type of illness behavior does not invariably occur in every patient with specific characteristics. It much more depends on the interaction between patient and doctor, as well as on the patient's interpretation of online information resources (2, 3, 7).

Robert Kellner analyzed research findings concerned with the treatment of patients with functional medical disorders, and identified some elements that could be associated with a more favorable prognosis (8). He then developed a psychotherapeutic approach for improving illness behavior and treating hypochondriacal fears and beliefs, defined as explanatory therapy (9). Such a method was subsequently validated in a controlled investigation (10) that was concerned with the most severe form of dysfunctional illness behavior, hypochondriasis. It consists of providing accurate information, clarification, teaching of the principles of selective perception (attention to one part of the body makes the patient more aware of sensations in that part of the body than in other parts), reassurance, and repetition (9, 10). Carlotta Belaise and I modified the protocol to increase endurance to withdrawal symptoms after discontinuation of antidepressants (11). The physician (whether the psychiatrist or the consultant internist) overseeing the procedure is encouraged to use some ingredients of explanatory therapy in his/her assessment sessions. The clinical psychologist or other qualified mental health worker performing the sequential psychotherapeutic approach may refer to the structured protocol that is specified below.

Explanatory therapy is the basic ingredient of the first module of the sequential psychotherapeutic approach that has been mentioned in the previous chapter. The entire strategy encompasses three modules that may have variable duration according to the individualized needs of the patient (see Figures 8.1 and 8.2, pp. 87 and 88). Patients are seen every 1 or 2 weeks for a number of sessions ranging from 16 to 24.

Components of Explanatory Therapy

This module, aimed at the tapering phase, may take place at the beginning of the sequential approach (see Figure 8.1, p. 87) or in the middle (see Figure 8.2, p. 88). In this latter case, tapering and discontinuation are postponed after CBT for anxiety disorders which had not been previously treated with psychotherapeutic interventions. The duration of the module is variable (from two to six weekly sessions) depending on the tapering method; in any event, elements of explanatory therapy are used and reiterated to the patient throughout the sequential approach.

Explanatory therapy should begin before tapering antidepressant medications. In the first session, patients are encouraged to keep a diary in which they list the most disturbing symptoms that occur from one session to the next, with a score for each symptom (from 0 to 100, where 100 is the most bothersome). In the diary, they also report the situations in which the most distressing moments occurred. As long as therapy progresses, patients are encouraged to write alternative interpretations of what they experience (Table 9.1). They are instructed to bring the diary to each visit.

Several types of feedback are provided by the therapist and are written in the diary. The first is concerned with accurate information. The planned method of discontinuation is detailed to the patient. There is no way we can predict whether withdrawal symptoms are going to take place, nor their modalities of onset, severity, and duration. Patients are informed that symptoms may start appearing during tapering and tend to have a peak 1–2 weeks after discontinuation. Withdrawal symptoms are new symptoms that may slowly subside within a month or may persist for a longer time (months). Development of the right attitude toward symptom perception (to be learned during psychotherapy) may hasten their disappearance (11). There is evidence from research in psychophysiology that accurate information about a threatening somatic sensation can influence several phenomena, including the severity of autonomic responses and subjective distress (8, 9).

An additional component involves clarification, both of the previous faulty communications with physicians and about the nature of the sensations that were experienced. Patients have generally not been warned about the dependence potential of antidepressant drugs and may develop strong feelings about it. The question then becomes "How can this happen?" I often use the "antibiotic paradox" as an example: the best agents for treating bacterial infection are also the best agents for selecting

Table 9.1 Example of the Antidepressant Drugs Tapering Diary

Situation	Symptoms and intensity (0–100)	Interpretation
I am at home trying to prepare my lessons for tomorrow and dinner for my family.	I am feeling bad, confused. I will not be able to accomplish anything. I am having electric shock sensations. My lesson will be a failure. Intensity: 70	Electric shock sensations are caused by lowering the dose of the drug. I had the other symptoms also before starting the medication. I should calm down and something will come out.

and propagating resistant strains, which persist in the environment even when exposure to the drug is stopped (12). Antidepressant medications may be life-saving, but they also have the potential for dependence.

A third essential component involves explaining that there is a strong tendency to pay attention to some parts of the body and to perceive threatening stimuli accordingly (selective perception). As an example, if one is anxious about the arrival of another person, one hears footsteps in the corridor, whereas if one does not have a reason for anxiety, the footsteps are not perceived (9). The vivid experience of withdrawal symptoms ("neuroemotions") is likely to trigger a state of selective perception.

Finally, Kellner emphasized the difficulties that patients may have in registering and retaining complex information (8, 9). As a result, repetition and reassurance are also another important therapeutic ingredient of explanatory therapy (e.g., "It is quite frequent to have these symptoms upon tapering or after discontinuation of this drug"; "It is not a relapse, but a withdrawal reaction"; "It is just a transient phase, soon it may be over") (11). The consultant internist, by performing a physical examination, may provide very effective reassurance that, in my clinical experience, is highly appreciated by patients.

Providing this type of feedback induces "mental lighting" in patients (11). "If I had not been told that the symptoms I was experiencing after discontinuing venlafaxine were to be expected and that eventually there could be light at the end of the tunnel, I would have killed myself, because the mental pain was unbearable" wrote Emma, the young patient described in Chapter 3, at the end of therapy. She told me: "I did not know where in the tunnel I was, only darkness back and ahead. But I had the feeling that you could see me progressing in the tunnel and that you knew my position." Actually, it is quite difficult to have such a clear vision, but I am glad that Emma perceived no doubt or indecision in me.

The sessions of explanatory therapy that follow the initial one deal with the patient's diary. The diary consists of three columns: one in which the patient describes the situation when the most distressing symptoms occur; another in which the distress and symptoms experienced are described; and a third in which the patient records their interpretation of these experiences (in some cases supplemented with comments from the therapist). The patient learns that not all symptoms that are experienced may be attributed to the antidepressants (clarification). Table 9.1 provides an example of the diary of a schoolteacher, Veronica, during citalopram tapering. The diary is important also when there are no immediate withdrawal symptoms upon tapering: symptoms may ensue with further tapering or after discontinuation, or may begin weeks or months after discontinuation.

Patients are encouraged to keep on doing life activities and to pay as little attention as possible to symptoms (11). There are days which are bad but, if patients try to react, the days get better. In patients with a passive attitude to life and plenty of opportunities for paying attention to their symptoms, activity scheduling may be prescribed. Some motivational elements are introduced, explaining the concept of behavioral toxicity (see Chapter 3). Patients are reminded that the drug had become toxic to them and that, in the long run, they will feel much better. If clinical phenomena related to oppositional tolerance (e.g., loss of efficacy, paradoxical effects) or major side effects (e.g., weight gain) occur, they may be used effectively to suggest the importance of ridding the body of the antidepressant and the potential harms of simply changing the type of antidepressant. Finally, some lifestyle suggestions are given (e.g., avoidance of alcohol, limited caffeine consumption, physical exercise, sleep hygiene, balanced diet). The structure of this first module is summarized in Box 9.1.

Moving Forward

The duration of the first module is very flexible, based on the modalities of tapering chosen and, especially, on the therapist's appraisal of the level of insight and the capacity of reaction of the patient. With the introduction of the diary, an important step is taken. In fact, keeping a diary of distress is in itself an important therapeutic ingredient linked to the role of self-disclosure (13). Pennebaker (14) pioneered the therapeutic use of the diary and developed a protocol for the disclosure of traumatic experiences in writing. An impressive body of experimental studies has indicated that, compared to neutral writing, expressing traumatic experiences by writing may improve the psychological status and physical health, and may enhance the immune function, with a reduction in autonomic nervous system activity (14). Further, the diary is the basic step of CBT and WBT. Its use in the first module thus facilitates the transition to the following steps of the therapeutic procedure.

Box 9.1 Goals of the First Therapeutic Module

1. Checking the general status of the patient
2. Listing new symptoms that have occurred, ranked according to the level of distress
3. Illustrating the various steps of the tapering procedure chosen
4. Keeping a diary related to the worst moments and situations
5. Reviewing the diary, with particular reference to the onset of withdrawal symptoms
6. Encouraging the patient to keep on tapering, and eventually discontinuing, the antidepressant
7. Providing accurate information, clarification, teaching of the principles of selective perception, reassurance, and repetition
8. Activity scheduling if necessary
9. Homework assignments
10. Lifestyle suggestions

References

1. Mechanic D: Sociological dimensions of illness behavior. Soc Sci Med 1995; 41:1207–16.
2. Cosci F, Fava GA: The clinical inadequacy of the DSM-5 classification of somatic symptoms and related disorders: an alternative trans-diagnostic model. CNS Spectrums 2016; 21:310–17.
3. Fava GA, Cosci F, Sonino N: Current psychosomatic practice. Psychother Psychosom 2017; 86:13–30.
4. Fava GA, Rafanelli C, Tomba E: The clinical process in psychiatry: a clinimetric approach. J Clin Psychiatry 2012; 73:177–84.
5. de las Cuevas, de Leon J: Reviving research on medication attitudes for improving pharmacotherapy. Psychother Psychosom 2017; 86:73–9.
6. Schweizer E, Rickels K, de Martinis N, Case G, Garcia-Espanha F: The effect of personality on withdrawal severity and taper outcome in benzodiazepine dependent patients. Psychol Med 1998; 28:713–20.
7. Cosci F, Guidi J: The role of illness behavior in the COVID-19 pandemic. Psychother Psychosom 2021; 90:156-9.
8. Kellner R: Somatization and Hypochondriasis. New York, Praeger, 1986.
9. Kellner R: Psychotherapeutic strategies in the treatment of psychophysiological disorders. Psychother Psychosom 1979; 32:91–100.

10. Fava GA, Grandi S, Rafanelli C, Fabbri S, Cazzaro M: Explanatory therapy in hypochondriasis. J Clin Psychiatry 2000; 61:317–22.
11. Fava GA, Belaise C: Discontinuing antidepressant drugs. Lessons from a failed trial and extensive clinical experience. Psychother Psychosom 2018; 87:257–67.
12. Levy SB: The Antibiotic Paradox: How Miracle Drugs Are Destroying the Miracle. New York, Plenum, 1992.
13. Guidi J, Brakemeier E-L, Bockting CLH, Cosci F, Cuijpers P, Jarrett RB, Linden M, Marks I, Peretti CS, Rafanelli C, Rief W, Schneider S, Schnyder U, Sensky T, Tomba E, Vazquez C, Vieta E, Zipfel S, Wright JH, Fava GA: Methodological recommendations for trials of psychological interventions. Psychother Psychosom 2018; 87:285–95.
14. Pennebaker JW: Writing about emotional experiences as a therapeutic process. Psychol Sci 1997; 8:162–6.

10

Second Psychotherapeutic Module

Cognitive-Behavioral Therapy

So far there have been very few applications of CBT to the discontinuation process of antidepressant medications. Scholten et al. (1) reported on the first RCT that attempted to use CBT to prevent relapse in patients with remitted anxiety disorder who discontinued antidepressant drugs (relapse prevention group), compared to treatment as usual. The patients who were assigned to CBT received eight group sessions for relapse prevention, targeting vulnerability factors and discontinuation symptoms. Antidepressant medications were tapered every 2 weeks within 4 months, according to a fixed schedule. In the control group (treatment as usual), tapering and discontinuation of antidepressant drugs were carried out without CBT, in individual sessions, according to the same schedule. Primary outcomes were occurrence/reoccurrence of any anxiety disorder or major depressive disorder. A secondary outcome was the success rate of discontinuation of antidepressant drugs. Seventy-three patients were enrolled. Over 16 months, there were no significant differences between the CBT group and the treatment-as-usual group in any of the primary and secondary outcome measures. Despite guidance, only 36% of all participants succeeded in discontinuing antidepressant medications, and only 28% did not have any recurrence. One patient committed suicide. The trial was stopped prematurely for ethical reasons and futility (1).

However, the trial was certainly not futile; it provided important insights (2). As the authors commented (1), the guideline recommendations for discontinuing antidepressants were found to be neither feasible nor effective in their sample. The investigators, while convinced they were applying the best evidence, found out that they had been simply misguided (2). Withdrawal symptoms and syndromes may occur during and despite slow tapering, do not magically vanish after a couple of weeks from discontinuation, and may persist for a long time, leading to postwithdrawal syndromes (2). In this trial (1), CBT was thus stopped when more was in fact needed. Further, withdrawal symptoms and syndromes were not adequately assessed and addressed; they might have been misidentified as the occurrence of an anxiety disorder (2).

Similar methodological problems affected another RCT of preventive cognitive therapy with antidepressant discontinuation during pregnancy (3). A modified version of CBT was associated with discontinuation of antidepressants and compared with continuation of this medication and care as usual (3). There were no significant differences between the two groups in terms of maternal risk of relapse into depression (3). Since, also in this case, withdrawal symptoms could have been misidentified as the occurrence of a depressive episode, the results cast serious doubts on the efficacy of antidepressant maintenance for preventing relapse in depression. The findings also indicate that discontinuation of antidepressant drugs is feasible during pregnancy.

There are two modalities of application of CBT in the sequential approach to discontinuing antidepressant medications. The strategy may be quite different in mood and anxiety disorders. In depression, there is the need for addressing residual symptomatology and cognitive styles that may, in the long run, lead to relapse (4, 5). In anxiety disorders, obsessive-compulsive illness, and post-traumatic stress disorder (PTSD) there is often the need to treat the original symptomatology that was only temporarily managed by pharmacological treatment. Not surprisingly, discontinuation of antidepressants in anxiety disorders entails a high likelihood of relapse (6). I will present the application of CBT as a second module (see Figure 8.1, p. 87), following explanatory therapy and antidepressant tapering (not necessarily full discontinuation), and before WBT. I will then describe the case when CBT becomes the first module and precedes explanatory therapy and medication tapering (see Figure 8.2, p. 88). An important clinical question is whether the patient received any effective, evidence-based psychotherapeutic treatment for anxiety, obsessions, and PTSD in addition to pharmacotherapy. If yes, what exactly was the protocol? The decision of using one module or the other relies completely on clinical judgment (in particular, the evaluation of the severity of disturbances of the original illness, which may be masked by the pharmacological treatment).

Cognitive-Behavioral Therapy Following Explanatory Therapy and Antidepressant Tapering: The Second Module

Keeping a structured diary of instances of distress (self-observation), as a source of awareness and reflection, is a basic cognitive behavioral technique (7–9). As Wright and associates remark, writing automatic thoughts down on paper (or on a computer or smartphone) "draws the patient's attention to important cognitions, provides a systematic method to practice identifying automatic thoughts, and often stimulates a sense of inquiry about the validity of the thoughts pattern. Just seeing thoughts written down on paper often sets off a spontaneous effort to revise or correct maladaptive cognitions" (9, p. 99). Schemas are organized, enduring representations of knowledge and experience, which guide the processing of information and interaction with life circumstances (7–9). For instance, depressed patients tend to have schemas that are characterized by themes of loss, failure, worthlessness, and rejection that lead to negative perceptions of themselves, the world, and the future (the cognitive triad) and to negative information-processing biases (7). Self-observation has a major role in behavioral therapy, with particular reference to homework exposure therapy of anxiety disorders (10). The central principle of treatment is to persuade the patient to re-enter the phobic situation and to remain there despite the ensuing anxiety (10). A structured diary of exposure tasks and subsequent accomplishments (how each exposure task went) is planned with the patient. The therapist reviews the diary with the patient and provides reassurance and guidance. The structured diary contains a mixture of negative and positive experiences, which should be properly modulated by the patient with the use of positive reinforcement (11). As a result, self-observation of distress and the building of a hierarchy of avoidances paves the way for cognitive behavioral intervention: schemas can be modified and avoidances can be overcome in the course of psychotherapy to achieve a functional role (7–11).

With the beginning of the second module, keeping a diary assumes a different connotation. The patient is instructed to record in a diary (Table 10.1) all episodes of distress which may ensue in the following 2 weeks. It is important to emphasize that distress (which is left unspecified) does not need to be prolonged, but may also be short-lived. Patients are also

Table 10.1 Example of Cognitive Restructuring from Veronica's Diary

Situation	Distress (intensity 0–100)	Negative automatic thoughts	Observer's interpretation
I am at home trying to prepare my lessons for tomorrow and dinner for my family.	I feel tense and anxious. (intensity level 60)	I am unable to accomplish anything. I am a total failure.	I am generally able to prepare decent lessons. This is just anxiety. If I try to calm down, I can make it.

instructed to compile a list of situations which elicit distress and/or tend to induce avoidance. Each situation should be rated on a 0–100 point scale (0 = no problem; 100 = panic, unbearable distress). Patients are required to bring the diary to the following visit.

A cognitive behavioral strategy is formulated. It may encompass both exposure and cognitive restructuring. Exposure consists of homework assignments only. An exposure strategy is planned with the patient, based on the list of situations outlined in the diary. The therapist writes an assignment for each day in the diary, following a graded exposure logic (10, 11). The patient assigns a score from 0 to 100 to each homework assignment. At the following visit, the therapist reassesses the completed homework and discusses the next steps and/or problems in compliance which may have ensued. Cognitive restructuring follows the format of Beck et al. (7, 8) and is based on the introduction of a rating of distress (0–100) and the concepts of automatic negative thoughts and of observer's interpretation, and relies on the use of macroanalysis (as described in Chapter 7). For instance, the situation reported by Veronica in Chapter 9 could be reformulated as in Table 10.1.

The problems which may be the object of cognitive restructuring strictly depend on the material offered by the patient. They may encompass anxious ideations, irritability, sleep problems, perception of diminished energy and concentration, residual hopelessness, re-entry problems (diminished functioning at work, avoidance, and procrastination), lack of assertiveness and self-care, perfectionism, and unrealistic self-expectations. All these symptoms may characterize the residual

---

Box 10.1 Goals of the Second Therapeutic Module

---

1. Checking the general status of the patient
2. Reviewing the diary, with particular reference to the trajectory of both withdrawal and affective symptoms
3. Identifying subclinical distress, avoidance, and residual symptoms
4. Providing information, reassurance, clarification, and repetition
5. Cognitive restructuring
6. Activity scheduling
7. Homework assignments
8. Lifestyle suggestions

---

phase of depressive illness (12). However, monitoring of withdrawal symptoms that may persist has to be maintained during the course of this second module. The psychotherapist should integrate the treatment of the original symptoms with the occurrence of new symptoms according to the patient's priorities and needs.

The structure of the second module is summarized in Box 10.1. It may extend over six to ten sessions, preferably every other week. Explanatory therapy is continued as needed. This second module can be accomplished by the psychologist, but a couple of assessments by the treating psychiatrist are essential. The medical consultant may be needed again.

Cognitive-Behavioral Therapy Preceding Explanatory Therapy and Antidepressant Tapering: The First Module

In a controlled trial (13), when CBT was performed in patients with panic disorder treated with antidepressant drugs, there was no significant difference in relapse between patients who discontinued versus those who continued medications (13). These findings were consistent with what we had observed in our open trial on discontinuing SSRIs in re-mitted patients with panic disorder and agoraphobia treated with behavioral methods (14): at 1-year follow-up there were plenty of withdrawal symptoms, but only in one case out of 20 patients was there a relapse of panic. When remission is obtained with CBT in anxiety disorders, there is strong a tendency to prolonged endurance (15), and this particularly applies to the effects of homework exposure in phobic disturbances (16, 17).

Despite treatment with antidepressant drugs, patients may still meet the diagnostic criteria for anxiety disorders and/or obsessive-compulsive disorder and/or PTSD (18), as was found to be frequently the case in clinical practice (16, 17). Or they may not meet specific criteria, but present with subclinical symptomatology, which has important implications. For instance, some subtle forms of avoidance may be associated with considerable functional impairment and invalidism ("I can go to that place, but only if ... ") (11). Once again, a clinimetric approach is essential (19). According to the psychometric model endorsed by DSM-5 (18), severity is determined by the number of symptoms, not by their intensity or quality, to the same extent that a score in a rating scale depends on the number of symptoms that are scored as present. Clinimetrics reflects the practice of clinical medicine, where not all symptoms are the same and should carry the same weight (19). The repeated use of macroanalysis with each assessment in the course of treatment, with attention to the longitudinal development and therapeutic response, may help differentiate comorbidity that wanes from disturbances that persist.

In my treatment manual for WBT (20), I have provided detailed protocols, session by session, of cognitive restructuring and homework exposure during cognitive behavioral therapy that may be followed by WBT sessions, according to the sequential integration of two psychotherapeutic strategies.

Moving Forward

A course of CBT may yield a wide range of responses. Not unlike drug treatment, psychotherapy in general practice may induce improvement in about half of cases, deterioration/worsening in a small subgroup, and no change in the remaining cases (21). The rationale of the sequential approach is that one course of treatment is unlikely to produce a solution to the complex disturbances that can be encountered in clinical practice (19, 22). The studies that used a sequential design clearly indicated that the level of remission that could be obtained by successful pharmacotherapy could be increased by a subsequent psychotherapeutic treatment (5, 22). Clinicians and researchers in clinical psychiatry often confound response to treatment with full recovery (23). Indeed, there is increasing evidence that full recovery can be reached only through interventions which facilitate progress toward achievement of euthymia (23, 24). Per Bech and I (25) have defined a state of euthymia as characterized by the features depicted in Figure 10.1. Jenny Guidi and I have recently developed guidelines for the clinical assessment of euthymia (23, 24). They encompass a structured interview, the Clinical Interview for Euthymia (with items covering positive affect, both polarities of psychological well-being

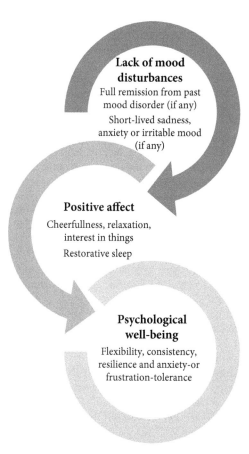

Figure 10.1 Clinical Features of Euthymia

dimensions, and information about flexibility, consistency, and resilience), and self-rating scales such as the Euthymia Scale (23–25).

As a result, the second full assessment after CBT (whether after the first or second sequential module) (see Figures 8.1 and 8.2, pp. 87 and 88) becomes of considerable importance, particularly if it is expanded to the assessment of euthymia. It may produce substantial changes in the macroanalysis, which is functional to the introduction of the third component of the psychotherapeutic module—WBT (20).

References

1. Scholten WD, Batelaan NM, van Oppen P, Smit JH, Hoogendoorn AW, van Megen HJGM, Cath DC, van Balkom AJLM: The efficacy of a group-CBT-relapse prevention program for remitted anxiety disorder patients who discontinue antidepressant medication: a randomized controlled trial. Psychother Psychosom 2018; 87:240–2.
2. Fava GA, Belaise C: Discontinuing antidepressants drugs. Lesson from a failed trial and extensive clinical experience. Psychother Psychosom. 2018; 87:257–67.
3. Molenaar NM, Brouwer ME, Burger H, Kamperman AM, Bergink V, Hoogendijk WJG, Williams AD, Bockting CLH, Lambregtse-van der Berg MP: Preventing cognitive therapy with antidepressant discontinuation during pregnancy: results from a randomized controlled trial. J Clin Psychiatry 2020; 81:1913099.
4. Fava GA: Sequential treatment: a new way of integrating pharmacotherapy and psychotherapy. Psychother Psychosom 1999; 68:227–9.
5. Guidi J, Tomba E, Fava GA: The sequential integration of pharmacotherapy and psychotherapy in the treatment of major depressive disorder: a meta-analysis of the sequential model and a critical review of the literature. Am J Psychiatry 2016; 173:128–37.
6. Batelaan NM, Bosman RC, Muntingh A, Scholten WD, Huijbregts KM, van Balkom AJLM: Risk of relapse after antidepressant discontinuation in anxiety disorders, obsessive-compulsive disorder, and post-traumatic stress disorder. BMJ 2017; 358:j3927.
7. Beck AT, Rush AJ, Shaw BF, Emery G: Cognitive Therapy of Depression. New York, Guilford, 1979.
8. Clark DA, Beck AT: Cognitive Therapy of Anxiety Disorders. Science and Practice. New York, Guilford, 2010.
9. Wright JH, Brown GK, Thase ME, Ramirez-Baco M: Learning Cognitive-Behavior Therapy. Second Edition. Arlington, VA, American Psychiatric Association Publishing, 2017.
10. Marks IM: Fears, Phobias and Rituals. New York, Oxford University Press, 1987.
11. Fava GA, Grandi S, Canestrari R, Grasso P, Pesarin F: Mechanisms of change of panic attacks with exposure treatment of agoraphobia. J Affect Disord 1991; 22: 65–71.

12. Guidi J, Tomba E, Cosci F, Park SK, Fava GA: The role of staging in planning psychotherapeutic interventions in depression. J Clin Psychiatry 2017; 78:456–63.

13. Schmidt NB, Wolllaway-Bickel K, Trakowski JH, Santiago HT, Vasey M: Antidepressant discontinuation in the context of cognitive behavioral treatment for panic disorder. Behav Res Ther 2002; 40:67–73.

14. Fava GA, Bernardi M, Tomba E, Rafanelli C: Effects of gradual discontinuation of selective serotonin reuptake inhibitors in panic disorder with agoraphobia. Int J Neuropsychopharmacol 2007; 10:835–8.

15. von Brachel R, Hirschfeld G, Berner A, Willutzki U, Teismann T, Cwik JC, Velten I, Schulte D, Margraf J: Long-term effectiveness of cognitive behavioral therapy in routine outpatient care: a 5- to 20-year follow-up. Psychother Psychosom 2019; 88:225–35.

16. Fava GA, Rafanelli C, Grandi S, Conti S, Ruini C, Mangelli L, Belluardo P: Long-term outcome of panic disorder with agoraphobia treated by exposure. Psychol Med 2001; 31:891–8.

17. Fava, GA, Grandi S, Rafanelli C, Ruini C, Conti S, Belluardo P: Long term outcome of social phobia treated by exposure. Psychol Med 2001; 31:899–905.

18. Diagnostic and Statistical Manual of Mental Disorders: Fifth Edition. DSM-5. Washington, DC, American Psychiatric Association, 2013.

19. Fava GA, Rafanelli C, Tomba E: The clinical process in psychiatry: a clinimetric approach. J Clin Psychiatry 2012; 73:177–84.

20. Fava GA: Well-Being Therapy: Treatment Manual and Clinical Applications. Basel, Karger, 2016.

21. Lambert MJ: Maximizing psychotherapy outcome beyond evidence-based medicine. Psychother Psychosom 2017; 86:80–9.

22. Guidi J, Fava GA: Sequential combination of pharmacotherapy and psychotherapy in major depressive disorder: a systematic review and meta-analysis. JAMA Psychiatry 2021; 78:261–9.

23. Fava GA, Guidi J: The pursuit of euthymia. World Psychiatry 2020; 19:40–50.

24. Guidi J, Fava GA: The emerging role of euthymia in psychotherapy research and practice. Clin Psychol Rev 2020; 82:101941.

25. Fava GA, Bech P: The concept of euthymia. Psychother Psychosom 2016; 85:1–5.

11

Third Psychotherapeutic Module

Well-Being Therapy

When I first saw Carol, she was a 34-year-old attorney suffering from panic attacks and agoraphobic avoidance that was she trying to hide as much as she could. Her panic attacks occurred with a frequency of a couple per month despite the use of sertraline (100 mg/day). She claimed sertraline—that she had been taking for 5 years (initially, 50 mg/day)—helped, but not to a satisfactory degree. I thought it was better to use the second option of sequential treatment (see Figure 8.2, p. 88), with CBT as a first therapeutic module, and to postpone any pharmacological change until after completion of CBT. Her agoraphobia was subtle, as often happens (1, 2): she could go to her office and to the tribunal every day, but refrained from doing anything different. She was single and living alone, something she disliked but had learned to live with. Carol reacted very well to a behavioral intervention I performed based on homework exposure (1, 2). There was a considerable decrease in anxiety and avoidance. However, she seemed to be in a sort of limbo, as depicted so well in the following description of the "antidepressed personality" written by a clinician in 1975: "Not anxious but not at ease; not incapable of working but not capable of working well; not tormented by children, but not able to enjoy them; willing to be made love to, but not actively loving; neither tense nor relaxed, neither ill nor well, more depressing than depressed" (3, p. 349).

When I voiced my intention to start tapering and discontinuing sertraline, Carol first rejected my proposal: "I am a weak person" she said. "I need the serotonin of the medication; without sertraline I would be depressed and hopeless." I thought of the spectacular achievements of propaganda that one of my teachers, Bish Lipowski, had anticipated more than three decades before:

Another current fad is to tell patients that they suffer from a chemical imbalance in the brain. The explanatory power of this statement is about the same order if you said to the patient: "You are alive." It confuses the distinction between etiology and correlation, and cause and mechanism, a common confusion in the field. It gives the patient a misleading impression that his or her imbalance is *the* cause of his or her illness, that it needs to be fixed by purely chemical means, that psychotherapy is useless and that personal efforts and responsibility have no part to play in getting better. (4, p. 252)

I tried to explain to her that sertraline was very unlikely to be more effective than placebo after 5 years, but I realized that my message was swimming against the tide of pharmaceutical propaganda. I added that if the positive effect of sertraline was doubtful, a detrimental effect was likely: a sense of numbing and/or of emotional blunting and/or of diminished affective responsiveness. The original observation of the "antidepressed personality" (3) has now in fact been substantiated by several research findings (5). This possibility motivated the attorney: "Pharmaceutical firms tend to hide side effects and it is clear that one never hears about them. Does it mean that I could feel better?". We agreed on tapering and discontinuing sertraline. We were blessed by some luck, since Carol did not develop any withdrawal symptoms. However, there was something else we had to work on, and I felt that WBT (6) was badly needed.

Shifting the Goal of Treatment:
Well-Being Therapy

In 1958, Marie Jahoda published an extraordinary book on positive mental health (7). She denied that "the concept of mental health can be usefully defined by identifying it with the absence of a disease. It would seem, consequently, to be more fruitful to tackle the concept of mental health in its more positive connotation, noting, however, that the absence of disease may constitute a necessary, but not sufficient, criterion for mental health" (7, pp. 14–15). She outlined criteria for positive mental health: autonomy (regulation of behavior from within); environmental mastery; satisfactory interactions with other people and the milieu; the individual's style and degree of growth, development, or self-actualization; and the attitudes of an individual toward his/her own self (self-perception/acceptance). The book indicated how mental health research was dramatically weighted on the side of psychological dysfunction. It took a long time (four decades) before such an imbalance started being corrected, as a result of the development of specific psychotherapeutic strategies, such as WBT (8). WBT can be differentiated from other psychotherapeutic approaches, including positive interventions, on the basis of the following features:

1. **Monitoring of psychological well-being in a diary** The main difference is that patients are encouraged to identify episodes of well-being and optimal experiences in a structured diary, and to set them in a situational context (6, 8). These contexts are characterized by the perception of high environmental challenges and environmental mastery, deep concentration, involvement, enjoyment, control of the situation, clear feedback on the course of activity, and intrinsic motivation (9). All other psychotherapeutic approaches focus on distress.

2. **Identification of low tolerance to well-being by seeking automatic thoughts** Once the instances of well-being are properly recognized, the patient is encouraged to identify thoughts and beliefs leading to premature interruption of well-being (automatic thoughts), as is performed in cognitive therapy (10). The trigger for self-observation is, however, different, being based on well-being instead of distress.

3. **Behavioral exposure** The therapist may also reinforce and encourage activities that are likely to elicit well-being and optimal experiences (e.g., assigning the task of undertaking particular pleasurable activities for a certain time each day). Meeting the challenge that optimal experiences may entail is emphasized, because it is through this challenge that growth and improvement of self can take place.

4. **Cognitive restructuring using specific psychological well-being models** The monitoring of the course of episodes of well-being allows the therapist to realize specific impairments or excessive levels in Jahoda's well-being dimensions (7), as categorized by Ryff (11).

The individual thus becomes able to readily identify moments of well-being, be aware of interruptions to well-being feelings (interfering thoughts and/or behaviors), utilize cognitive behavioral techniques to address these interruptions, and pursue optimal experiences.

5. **Individualized and balanced focus** Patients are not simply encouraged to pursue the highest possible levels in psychological well-being in all dimensions, as is found to be the case in most positive interventions, but also to obtain a balanced functioning, subsumed under the rubric of euthymia (see Figure 10.1, p. 115). A state of euthymia could be different from one individual to another, depending on factors such as personality traits, social roles, and cultural and social contexts (12, 13).

WBT is thus a short-term psychotherapeutic strategy that emphasizes self-observation of psychological well-being, with the use of a structured diary, cognitive restructuring of interfering thoughts and/or behaviors through cognitive behavioral techniques, and homework assignments (e.g., pursuing optimal experiences) (6). WBT has been validated in a number of RCTs. It has been used mainly in sequential combination after CBT, and was found to be superior to active control conditions in depression (14–17), cyclothymic disorder (18), and in the setting of depression and demoralization after acute coronary events (19). A dismantling study that was performed in generalized anxiety disorder (20), where patients were randomly assigned to eight sessions of CBT or the sequential administration of four sessions of CBT followed by four sessions of WBT, suggested that an increased level of recovery could be obtained with the addition of WBT to CBT. It should be noted, however, that the sequential combination of CBT and WBT (with the addition of explanatory therapy) that is described here has not been specifically tested with a properly designed and performed RCT in the specific setting of antidepressant discontinuation, but only within the sequential model applied to recurrent depression (12, 13).

WBT introduces a shift in self-observation. Patients are now asked to report in the diary the circumstances surrounding their episodes of well-being and optimal experiences, rated on a 0–100 scale, with 0 being the absence of well-being and 100 the most intense well-being that could be

Table 11.1 The Bipolar Nature of the Dimensions of Psychological Well-Being

Impaired level	Balanced level	Excessive level
ENVIRONMENTAL MASTERY		
The person has difficulties in managing situations in everyday life; he/she feels unable to improve things; he/she is unaware of opportunities.	The person has a sense of competence in managing the environment; he/she makes good use of surrounding opportunities; he/she is able to choose what is more suitable to his/her personal needs.	The person is constantly looking for difficult situations to be handled; he/she is unable to savor positive emotions and leisure time; he/she is too engaged in work or family activities.
PERSONAL GROWTH		
The person has a sense of being stuck; he/she lacks perception of improvement over time; he/she feels bored and uninterested in life.	The person has a sense of continued development; he/she sees self as growing and improving; he/she is open to new experiences.	The person is unable to elaborate past negative experiences; he/she cultivates illusions that clash with reality; he/she has unrealistic standards and goals.
PURPOSE IN LIFE		
The person lacks a sense of meaning in life; he/she has few goals or purposes and lacks a sense of direction.	The person has goals in life and feels there is meaning to his/her present and past life.	The person has unrealistic expectations and hopes; he/she is constantly dissatisfied with his/her performance and is unable to recognize failures.
AUTONOMY		
The person is overconcerned with others' expectations and evaluations; he/she relies on the judgment of others to make important decisions.	The person is independent and able to resist social pressures; he/she is able to regulate behavior and self by personal standards.	The person is unable to get along with other people, to work in a team, or to learn from others; he/she is unable to ask for advice or help when needed.
SELF-ACCEPTANCE		
The person feels dissatisfied with self and/or disappointed with what has occurred in his/her past life; he/she wishes to be different.	The person accepts his/her good and bad qualities, and feels positive about his/her past life.	The person has difficulties in admitting his/her own mistakes; he/she attributes all problems to others' faults.

(cont.)

Table 11.1 *Continued*

Impaired level	Balanced level	Excessive level
POSITIVE RELATIONS WITH OTHERS		
The person has very few close, trusting relationships with others; he/she finds it difficult to be open.	The person has trusting relationships with others; he/she is concerned about the welfare of others; he/she understands the "give and take" of human relationships.	The person sacrifices his/her needs and well-being for those of others; low self-esteem and sense of worthlessness induce excessive readiness to forgive.

experienced. Review of the diary allows the identification of impaired or excessive dimensions of well-being, according to the conceptual framework by Jahoda (7), using Ryff's categorization of dimensions (11), as illustrated in Table 11.1.

Characteristics of well-being are, in fact, neither positive nor negative (6). Use of the well-being diary, together with cognitive restructuring and exposure homework, may provide a different outlook to patients. Many patients, as in the case of Carol at the beginning of this chapter, are convinced that they cannot make it without antidepressant drugs because they are weak and vulnerable. Negative cognitive schemas concerned with environmental mastery ("I cannot function without antidepressants") and purpose in life ("There is no life after antidepressants") can emerge, but through WBT they can also be corrected. The dimension of personal growth may be very important in making the person aware of some positive changes, both in terms of reduction of withdrawal symptomatology in the course of time ("Brain zaps still occur, but are less frequent now than before, and other symptoms have decreased as well") and of re-experience/discovery of positive emotions that were numbed or anesthetized by antidepressant drugs (3, 5). "I feel that now I am more alive" Carol said "both in what is good and bad in my life." Table 11.2 is taken from the diary of Veronica, the schoolteacher I have referred to in Chapters 9 and 10.

Further imbalances in other dimensions of psychological well-being may occur. The patient may attribute all of his/her problems to the medications and does not admit that there were problems also before (excessive self-acceptance), may have impairments in autonomy ("I always

Table 11.2 Example of the Well-Being Diary

Situation	Well-being (intensity 0–100)	Interrupting thoughts or behaviors	Observer
In class, I was able to handle a very disturbing student.	I am feeling very good and proud. (Intensity score 70)	It is just a single episode. It does not mean anything.	It is not a single episode. I am getting more and more in control, even though I no longer take antidepressants.

have to depend on someone or something; I cannot do anything by myself"), and may underestimate his/her potential in terms of relationships with others ("No one could stand me, and without antidepressants I am unbearable").

The structure and goals of the third module are described in Box 11.1. As was found to be the case in the second module, the psychological work needs to be linked with psychiatric and medical follow-up.

Box 11.1 Goals of the Third Therapeutic Module

1. Checking the general status of the patient and the potential development of a persistent postwithdrawal disorder
2. Introducing the change in focus of psychotherapy (well-being instead of distress)
3. Using the well-being diary: self-monitoring of instances of well-being, thoughts, and/or behaviors leading to premature interruption, with the introduction of the observer's column (cognitive restructuring)
4. Introducing the concept of optimal experiences and their pursuit
5. Making the patient aware of improvements in withdrawal symptomatology
6. Activity scheduling
7. Homework assignments
8. Lifestyle suggestions

The Importance of Follow-Up Evaluations

Follow-up evaluations are crucial after conclusion of the therapeutic modules. The outcomes can be so different. There are patients like Carol who did not have any withdrawal symptomatology, did not need clonazepam at all, and had an important shift to euthymia. The psychotherapeutic experience prompted major changes in her life: she realized that the firm she was working in did not allow her to grow professionally, and moved to a more challenging, but rewarding position (in professional terms; regrettably, very little changed in financial terms). Carol started dating a man after many years. Conversely, Veronica went through a persistent, painful, and frustrating postwithdrawal disorder (protraction of withdrawal syndrome) which, however, faded in a year. Emma quit her job and moved to another country to enter a prestigious PhD program on the subject she always liked, but continued to have brain zaps and genital pain at a 3-year follow-up, even though with lower intensity and frequence. There are patients who are unable to discontinue antidepressants and give up, or who discontinue them but want to go back (as did one patient who, after 20 years' treatment with paroxetine, was able to discontinue but then wanted to go back onto it, without the results she had before, and who cursed my intervention and meeting me). Finally, there are patients who relapse upon tapering and/or discontinuation of antidepressant drugs (and this particularly applies to anxiety disorders), even though all pharmacological and psychotherapeutic procedures were endorsed. They simply can no longer make it without antidepressant medications.

RCTs comparing different strategies, with long-term follow-ups, may provide essential data on the benefits, likelihood of responsiveness, and disadvantages of different approaches. We need neurobiological investigations that may shed some light on why, with the same treatment for the same duration of time, certain patients develop withdrawal syndromes and others do not. This should take place both at preclinical (21) and clinical levels. Longitudinal studies exploring the occurrence, clinical features, and neurobiological correlates of persistent postwithdrawal disorders are also a priority. Such studies may clarify the relationships between withdrawal syndromes and other manifestations of behavioral toxicity (e.g., refractoriness, loss of clinical effects), as well as distinguish whether a specific treatment worsened the symptoms or was simply in-effective, and whether the clinical picture would have deteriorated irre-spective of treatment.

WBT is in line with the concept that recovery is a one-way street, as I il-lustrated in Chapter 4. One should not be thinking of going back to a pre-treatment position. Flourishing and resilience can be promoted, leading to a positive evaluation of one's self, a sense of continuous growth and development, the belief that life is purposeful and meaningful, quality relations with others, the capacity to manage effectively one's life, and a sense of self-determination. A decreased vulnerability to depression and anxiety has been demonstrated after WBT in mood and anxiety disorders (14–20), and this may suggest a lower likelihood to use antidepressant drugs in the future. Once again, this hypothesis should be tested in RCTs. According to the oppositional model of tolerance, patients who develop behavioral toxicity, such as withdrawal symptoms, are at greater risk of developing depressive relapse (see Chapter 4) and thus need close follow-up assessments (every 6 or 12 months).

References

1. Marks IM: Fears, Phobias and Rituals. New York, Oxford University Press, 1987.
2. Fava GA, Grandi S, Canestrari R, Grasso P, Pesarin F: Mechanisms of change of panic attacks with exposure treatment of agoraphobia. J Affect Disord 1991; 22:65-71.
3. Mayer DY: Psychotropic drugs and the 'antidepressed' personality. Br J Med Psychol 1975; 48:349-57.
4. Lipowski ZJ: Psychiatry: mindless or brainless, both or neither? Can J Psychiatry 1989; 35:249-54.
5. Goodwin GM, Price J, De Bodinat C, Laredo J: Emotional blunting with antide-pressant treatments. J Affect Disord 2017; 221:31-5.
6. Fava GA: Well-Being Therapy: Treatment Manual and Clinical Applications. Basel, Karger, 2016.
7. Jahoda M: Current Concepts of Positive Mental Health. New York, Basic Books, 1958.
8. Fava GA, Rafanelli C, Cazzaro M, Conti S, Grandi S: Well-being therapy: a novel psychotherapeutic approach for residual symptoms of affective disorders. Psychol Med 1998; 28:475-80.
9. Csikszentmihalyi M, Csikszentmihalyi I: Optimal Experience. Psychological Studies of Flow in Consciousness. New York, NY, Cambridge University Press, 1988.

10. Wright JH, Brown GK, Thase ME, Ramirez-Baco M: Learning Cognitive-Behavior Therapy. Second Edition. Arlington, VA, American Psychiatric Association Publishing, 2017.
11. Ryff CD: Psychological well-being revisited. Psychother Psychosom 2014; 83:10–28.
12. Guidi J, Fava GA: The emerging role of euthymia in psychotherapy research and practice. Clin Psychol Rev 2020; 82:101941.
13. Fava GA, Guidi J: The pursuit of euthymia. World Psychiatry 2020; 19:40–50.
14. Fava GA, Rafanelli C, Grandi S, Conti S, Belluardo P: Prevention of recurrent depression with cognitive behavioral therapy: preliminary findings. Arch Gen Psychiatry 1998; 55:816–20.
15. Fava GA, Ruini C, Rafanelli C, Finos L, Conti S, Grandi S: Six-year outcome of cognitive behavior therapy for prevention of recurrent depression. Am J Psychiatry 2004; 161:1872–6.
16. Stangier U, Hilling C, Heidenreich T, Risch AK, Barocka A, Schlösser R, Kronfeld K, Ruckes C, Berger H, Röschke J, Weck F, Volk S, Hambrecht M, Serfling R, Erkwoh R, Stirn A, Sobanski T, Hautzinger M: Maintenance cognitive-behavioral therapy and manualized psychoeducation in the treatment of recurrent depression: a multicenter prospective randomized controlled study Am J Psychiatry 2013; 170:624–32.
17. Kennard BD, Emslie GJ, Mayes TL, Nakonezny PA, Jones JM, Foxwell AA, King J: Sequential treatment with fluoxetine and relapse-prevention CBT to improve outcomes in pediatric depression. Am J Psychiatry 2014; 171:1083–90.
18. Fava GA, Rafanelli C, Tomba E, Guidi J, Grandi S: The sequential combination of cognitive behavioral treatment and well-being therapy in cyclothymic disorder. Psychother Psychosom 2011; 80:136–43.
19. Rafanelli C, Gostoli S, Buzzichelli S, Guidi J, Sirri L, Gallo P, Marzola E, Bergerone S, De Ferrari GM, Roncuzzi R, Di Pasquale G, Abbate Daga G, Fava GA: Sequential combination of cognitive-behavioral treatment and well-being therapy in depressed patients with acute coronary syndromes. A randomized controlled trial (TREATED-ACS Study). Psychother Psychosom 2020; 89:345–56.
20. Fava GA, Ruini C, Rafanelli C, Finos L, Salmaso L, Mangelli L, Sirigatti S: Well-being therapy of generalized anxiety disorder. Psychother Psychosom 2005; 74:26–30.
21. Zabegalov KN, Kolesnikova TO, Khatsko SL, Volgin AD, Yakovlev OA, Amstislavskaya TG, Alekseeva PA, Meshalkina DA, Friend AJ, Bao W, Demin KA, Gainetdinov RR, Kalueff AV: Understanding antidepressant discontinuation syndrome (ADS) through preclinical experimental models. Eur J Pharmacol. 2018; 829:129–40.

12

Prevention of Dependence and Withdrawal Symptomatology Caused by Antidepressant Medications

Antidepressant prescribing has increased dramatically, year after year, since the introduction of SSRIs and SNRIs. For instance, it has been calculated that more than 10% of adults in England are now taking antidepressant drugs for depression/anxiety/distress, with a median length of treatment of more than 2 years (1). This is expected to increase to an even higher rate after the COVID-19 pandemic (though at the time of writing, this has still to be verified). In the previous chapters, I have tried to summarize what can be done, on the basis of the available literature and my clinical experience, to help those people who want or need to discontinue antidepressant drugs. Dependence on, and an inability to stop taking antidepressants represent a major, silent health emergency that has not received appropriate attention from national health services and research agencies throughout the world. New service modalities need to be established (see Chapter 6), and the clinical phenomena related to tapering and discontinuing antidepressant drugs should become a top priority for medical research and the mental health field.

The problems and difficulties that patients encounter in discontinuing antidepressant medications, and the increasing awareness of their long-term complications, alert us to the need of preventing the occurrence of dependence, with its ensuing problems of withdrawal symptomatology. Preventive efforts encompass strategies to reduce initial prescribing of antidepressants, clinical decisions that are likely to trigger cascade iatrogenesis, and the long-term use of these medications.

Reducing Initial Prescriptions

Bernard J. Carroll warned about the inappropriate use of antidepressant drugs nearly four decades ago: "We strongly suspect that many patients who are simply unhappy or dysphoric receive these drugs, with predictable consequences in terms of morbidity from side effects, mortality from overdose, economic waste, and irrational, unproductive clinical management" (2, p. 169). An increasing amount of research has substantiated the inappropriate use of antidepressants in patients who are simply going through some stressful circumstances or have some minor symptoms that do not reach the threshold of diagnostic criteria (1). We seem to have forgotten that the primary indication for the use of antidepressants is the treatment of a major depressive disorder, where they may be life-saving drugs. Their overall effectiveness has been inflated by selective reporting of positive trials (3). Antidepressant medications are unlikely to be better than placebo in mild or minor depression (4, 5). Even when a certain degree of severity is established, the clinical threshold provided by diagnostic criteria can be lowered by the presence of anxiety disturbances; anxious depression is less likely to respond to antidepressant medications compared to non-anxious depression (6).

If a patient suffers from severe depression, there is little doubt that pharmacotherapy may yield substantial benefits, even though, of course, response may vary from patient to patient. However, if symptoms of mild or moderate intensity are present, the benefits may be minimal or nonexistent (4, 5). Particularly in primary care and general hospital settings, a significant proportion of patients, and even those who initially fulfill diagnostic criteria for a major depressive episode, will improve without treatment after a few weeks or when they are discharged from the hospital (1, 7). Unless depression is severe and with suicidal ideations, a reasonable strategy is to postpone prescribing an antidepressant drug and to see the patient again after a couple of weeks (8). The neglect of the clinical phenomena related to tolerance may urge the clinician to give it a trial—a position that does not reflect the evidence in the field on the effectiveness of placebo and the likelihood that depressive symptoms remit with non-specific ingredients (9).

Kendrick (1) suggested that antidepressant medications are best avoided at the initial consultation for problems of depression not reaching the severity of diagnostic criteria, and drugs are justified only if subthreshold symptoms do not respond to a psychosocial intervention, or the patient is at risk of developing more severe depression in light of previous episodes and their prodromal symptomatology, or the patient suffers from recurrent mood disorders. If the prescription of antidepressant drugs were limited to these exceptions and clear-cut cases of major or persistent depressive disorders, we could certainly witness a welcome decrease in their use.

Another area where antidepressant medications should be used sparingly is with anxiety disorders. In the past two decades, a progressive change in prescribing patterns from BZs to second-generation antidepressants for anxiety disorders, obsessive-compulsive disorder, and PTSD has been observed (10). In a systematic review (11), no consistent evidence emerged supporting the advantage of using antidepressants over BZs in treating anxiety disorders. Indeed, BZs showed fewer treatment withdrawals and adverse events than antidepressant medications (11). In panic disorder with and without agoraphobia, BZ treatment was more effective in reducing the number of panic attacks than antidepressants (11). If we compare the side effects of SSRIs and BZs for panic disorder, as was done in a recent systematic review (12), the comparison is clearly in favor of BZs.

There were commercial reasons for this shift. BZs, because of their widespread use and limited cost, were a major obstacle to the introduction of the new antidepressants for anxiety disorders. A commercial war was thus started: the dependence potential of BZs was dramatized and their prescription was hindered in all possible ways, despite the clinical value of this class of medication (13). Physicians learned that BZs were bad and could cause dependence, whereas antidepressants were devoid of such effects. However, in due course, after their introduction, more pronounced problems occurred with most of the newer antidepressants (see Chapters 2 and 3). It would seem that, with both types of drugs, withdrawal reactions and postwithdrawal syndromes may ensue, despite slow tapering. Yet, even though loss of clinical effect and paradoxical reactions may occur with long-term treatment with BZs, other vulnerabilities that have been described with antidepressant drugs (resistance, switch to mania or hypomania, refractoriness) are unlikely to occur with them (14).

The use of antidepressant medications may be justified when a major depressive episode is associated with an anxiety disorder. In all other cases, treatment with antidepressants should be carefully considered and restricted to cases where psychotherapeutic strategies are not available or effective, or BZs have failed to provide adequate relief. It should also be remembered that BZs were found to be effective in anxious and mild depression (15).

The various types of BZ may differ in their side-effect profile: rebound anxiety, withdrawal syndromes, and dependence appear to be greater with those agents with a short- to intermediate-elimination half-life than those with a long half-life (13). There are major clinical differences between BZs based on the joint consideration of relative lipid solubility, binding affinity, and half-life (13). Drugs like alprazolam and triazolam, which have very high lipid solubility, are associated with higher dependence liability, cognitive impairment, and anterograde amnestic effects (13, 16). Conversely, BZs with low affinity for the BZ receptor and lipid solubility, such as clonazepam, appear to be associated with less dependence liability and amnestic potential (13, 16). Such characteristics are quite different from the conventional beta half-life (the rate of decline in the blood due to elimination or conjugation) (17).

Regardless of the type of medication, however, pharmacological therapy cannot be the first-line treatment of anxiety disorders, obsessive-compulsive disorder, and PTSD, due to the efficacy of psychotherapeutic approaches, with particular reference to CBT (18), and their enduring effects, as discussed in Chapter 10. Use of antidepressant medications, instead of BZs, may indeed yield long-term catastrophic results in anxiety disturbances, particularly in children and adolescents. Let us just think of one form of behavioral toxicity (behavioral activation and switch into bipolar disorder) that occurs significantly more in children than adults when antidepressants are used for anxiety (19), and is probably only the tip of the iceberg of phenomena related to the oppositional model of tolerance (see Chapters 3 and 4). One should also be concerned about young patients who start taking antidepressant drugs for anxiety disorders and prolong this treatment indefinitely without undergoing any form of psychotherapy. What will be the long-term outcome of their disturbances? Will tolerance develop and trigger deterioration and refractoriness?

Finally, there is increasing evidence suggesting the need to avoid or limit the use of antidepressant medications in bipolar disorder (8). Unfortunately, however, recognition of these mood disorders appears to be difficult in the primary care setting, since it requires expert interviewing.

Incorporating the Iatrogenic Perspective into Clinical Decisions

Clinical decisions concerned with the application of knowledge to the individual patient need to be placed in the framework of potential benefits of treatment, likelihood of responsiveness to the therapeutic option, and vulnerability to adverse effects (8, 20). However, if one perspective (vulnerability to adverse effects) is minimized or even denied, the ensuing balance is affected. We may then believe that a trial with antidepressant medications is always worth doing: what do we have to lose? As I have illustrated in Chapter 2, withdrawal reactions have been renamed as discontinuation syndromes, as if they were different from what was known about other psychotropic drugs, such as BZs. Both physicians and patients were taught that the problem could have appeared only with abrupt discontinuation of antidepressant drugs and that, if symptoms arose, they had to be considered signs of relapse, with prompt re-administration of the medication (21). The growth of EBM, with its emphasis on benefits and liability to pharmaceutical influences through vested meta-analyses, provided an ideal ground for minimizing the role of iatrogenic effects (22). As a result, the prescribing physician is driven by guidelines to an overestimated consideration of potential benefits, little attention to the likelihood of responsiveness, and neglect of potential vulnerabilities to the adverse effects of treatment (22). This applies to antidepressants as well as other medications, such as anti-inflammatory drugs and statins (23).

An illustration of the importance of the iatrogenic perspective for a correct balancing comes from the clinical situations subsumed under the rubric of treatment-resistant depression. Definitions of treatment resistance in depression are generally based on failure to respond to a trial with antidepressant drugs or, with a more stringent specification, on insufficient responses to at least two courses of adequate treatment (24).

Adequate drug treatment is generally defined as the use of antidepressant drugs at doses significantly superior to placebo in double-blind studies administered continuously for a minimum duration of 6 weeks (24). However, current conceptualizations of treatment resistance focus on the characteristics of the patient (whether neurobiological assets, or symptoms, or psychiatric comorbidity) for the lack of effectiveness of antidepressant drugs and omit any reference to the potential iatrogenic effects of treatment (25). It is as if, in the field of infectious disease, treatment resistance was conceptualized independently of previous use of antibiotics.

The ill-defined concept of treatment resistance is thus based on the untested assumption that treatment was right in the first place, and failure to respond is shifted upon patients' characteristics. Labeling what falls outside the limits of responsiveness as resistance is questionable. For instance, anxious depression is less likely to respond to antidepressant drugs compared to non-anxious depression (6). In a sample characterized by anxiety and depression of mild severity, we can shift into the realm of resistance what is simply the result of a treatment that has limited efficacy. Similar considerations may apply to the limited effectiveness of novel antidepressants (26). Treatment resistance thus calls for switching and augmentation, despite the lack of long-term efficacy of these procedures (27, 28). Indeed, such pharmacological manipulations may trigger cascade iatrogenesis, instead of reconsideration of the process in treatment selection (25).

Resistance to re-challenge, loss of clinical effects, paradoxical reactions, and withdrawal and postwithdrawal syndromes tend to cluster, and may share a common mechanism that has been subsumed under the rubric of oppositional model of tolerance (see Chapter 4). Very seldom are these phenomena considered in the clinical process. We have previously seen how treatment outcome is the cumulative result of the interaction of several classes of variables that may be therapeutic or counter-therapeutic (see Figure 5.1, p. 52). In certain patients, their interactive combination may lead to clinical improvement, whereas in other cases, it may produce no effect, and, in a third group, it may lead to worsening of the condition. Looking for counter-therapeutic ingredients is an important and yet neglected issue when treatments have failed.

Illness behavior—in its experiential, cognitive, and behavioral aspects—is an additional important source of difference in therapeutic outcomes (29). For instance, in psychiatric practice, one can observe that certain types of patient seem to antagonize drug effects, whether this is due to psychological reactance (a motivational force that leads individuals to fear loss of control), the balance between internal and external health-control beliefs, or illness behavior (25, 30). Such clinical phenomena can be easily found in the setting of personality disturbances (31). Yet they do not invariably occur in every patient with certain characteristics, because they depend on the interaction between patient and doctor. Other counter-therapeutic elements stem from dysfunctional cognitive schemas: prospective studies have shown that more negatively biased cognitive schemas are associated with a worse clinical course and more severe symptomatology (32). Conversely, the presence of unaffected areas of psychological well-being may predict a more favorable clinical course (32). There is a wide variation in the characteristics of illness behavior in depressed patients (33) and in the response of both positive and negative schemas to treatment (32). Both illness behavior and dysfunctional cognitive schemas may antagonize pharmacological treatment (34), as the following retrospective consideration of a patient illustrates:

> When I first saw you doctor, I had consulted an endless number of specialists, who had labeled me as a hopeless case of treatment resistance. I had the feeling that no one did really understand the pain I had inside and simply dismissed me with some different medications. I ended up convincing myself I was hopeless, but an internal anger kept me reacting and looking for help. I realize now that my attitude of those days could neutralize any treatment.

Iatrogenic factors are generally neglected in consideration of treatment-resistant depression, and such an omission may only lead to the use of more and more medications, in a tragic cascade.

Shortening Treatment Duration

Studies using routinely available data have indicated that the main reason use of antidepressant medications has increased so much in recent years is the increase in treatment duration (1). Lack of proper guidance for primary care physicians on the duration of treatment, lack of verification of the needs of therapy, and time constraints in follow-up appointments of specialists (medication checks) are three frequent additions (1) to the difficulties and insufficient directions that patients encounter when they attempt to discontinue antidepressants on their own (see Chapter 2). Indeed, the success rate of discontinuing antidepressants in primary care, with tapering guidance, was found to be less than 10% (35).

There is high inter-individual variability of the time that is necessary to recover from a depressive episode. At least 6 months of drug treatment appear to be necessary for most patients to reach a satisfactory level of remission (36). This time can be shortened to 3 months before tapering if the sequential combination of pharmacotherapy and psychotherapy is employed (37, 38). As I discussed in previous chapters, the sequential design is an intensive, two-stage approach, where one type of treatment (psychotherapy) is employed to improve symptoms which another type of treatment (pharmacotherapy) was unable to affect. This approach seeks to use psychotherapeutic strategies in a manner that is most likely to achieve a more pervasive recovery, by addressing residual symptomatology and by making a specific and substantial contribution to the patient's well-being (37, 38).

There are two essential models of sequential treatment: one in which pharmacotherapy is continued; the other where it is tapered and discontinued. Since there are no significant differences between the two approaches as to relapse rate (37, 38), one can conclude that maintenance pharmacotherapy is a redundant therapeutic ingredient for many (but not all) patients. Further, the literature indicates that, unlike in primary care (35), discontinuation of antidepressants appears to be feasible here (37, 38) and the success rate may reach 95% of patients. Indeed, the sequential approach that I have outlined in Chapters 8 to 11 is based on such evidence.

The available literature, however, should be interpreted with caution, in view of several issues. First, the data only reflect a general tendency, and there are many patients who simply cannot make it without antidepressant medications (35). Second, several of these studies were based on patients who had responded to initial treatment; patients at high risk may have dropped out early. Third, the investigations that used a sequential design had relapse-prevention purposes (39) and did not specifically address populations of patients who wanted to discontinue medications. Finally, a limiting step in translating the findings of RCTs that used the sequential model into practice is the fact that it requires, beyond just the automatic sequence of pharmacotherapy and psychotherapy, a number of clinical expert features (40), as detailed in Box 12.1, and these may not be easily available. I have outlined most of these features in the previous chapters. One (individualized focus) is worth detailing here. Therapeutic targets are not predetermined, but depend on the response of patients to the first course of treatment, such as the amount of residual symptomatology (41), the presence of occupational disability (42), the level of social functioning (43), and lifestyle (44). These strategies, whether psychotherapeutic or pharmacological, may be chosen on the basis of the target and not as a predefined option.

Since incomplete recovery from the first lifetime major depressive episode was found to predict a chronic course of illness during a 12-year prospective naturalistic follow-up (45), the sequential approach appears to be particularly indicated when major depression occurs for the first time in the patient's life.

Box 12.1 Specific Clinical Features for Best Applying the Sequential Model in Recurrent Depression

- Careful assessment of the patient, after adequate duration of antidepressant drug treatment (2–3 months), using clinimetric methods including staging and macroanalysis
- Use of individual or group psychotherapeutic strategies that depart from standard cognitive-behavioral measures and are geared to residual symptoms, and/or lifestyle modification, and/or well-being
- Individualized focus
- Careful reassessment of the patient, after second-line treatment has been completed and at subsequent points in time, with clinimetric methods for discriminating relapse from withdrawal symptomatology
- Multidisciplinary treatment team

On Miseducation and the Need of a
Counter-Culture

We have seen that if we try to balance the potential benefits of antidepressant medications with their likelihood of responsiveness and adverse
events, a rational use of antidepressants consists in targeting their application only to the most severe and persistent cases of depression, limiting
their use to the shortest possible time, and reducing their utilization in
anxiety disorders, unless a major depressive disorder is present or other
treatments have been ineffective (8). The importance of a psychotherapeutic approach for addressing residual symptoms with enduring effects
has also been emphasized. However, these indications run counter to
the type of information a physician or other health worker is likely to receive (46).

We have also seen that managing antidepressant discontinuation and
preventing the onset of dependence by reducing and shortening the
use of antidepressant drugs require a psychiatric approach that departs
from standard, mainstream trends and tendencies. It calls for a revolu-
tion in our way of thinking, assessing, and treating mood and anxiety
disorders.

References

1. Kendrick T: Strategies to reduce use of antidepressants. Br J Clin Pharmacol 2021;
   87:23–33.
2. Carroll BJ: Neurobiologic dimensions of depression and mania. In: Angst J (ed).
   The Origins of Depression: Current Concepts and Approaches. Berlin, Springer-
   Verlag, 1983, pp. 163–86.
3. Turner EH, Matthews AM, Linardatos E, Tell RA, Rosenthal R: Selective publication of antidepressants trials and its influence on apparent efficacy. N Engl J Med
   2008; 358:252–60.
4. Paykel ES, Hollyman JA, Freeling P, Sedgwick P: Predictors of therapeutic benefit
   from amitriptyline in mild depression. J Affect Disord 1988; 14:83–95.
5. Braillon A, Lexchin J, Noble JH, Menkes D, M'Sahli L, Fierlbeck K, Blumsohn A,
   Naudet F: Challenging the promotion of antidepressants for non-severe depression. Acta Psychiatr Scand 2019; 139:294–5.
6. Fava M, Rush J, Alpert JE, Balasubramani GK, Wisniewski SR, Carmin CN, Biggs
   MM, Zisook S, Leuchter A, Howland R, Warden D, Trivedi MH: Difference in
   treatment outcome in outpatients with anxious versus nonanxious depression.
   Am J Psychiatry 2008; 165:342–51.

7. Fava GA, Sonino N: Depression associated with medical illness. CNS Drugs 1996; 5:175–89.
8. Fava GA: Rational use of antidepressant drugs. Psychother Psychosom 2014; 83:197–204.
9. Rutherford B, Roose SP: A model of placebo response in antidepressant clinical trials. Am J Psychiatry 2013; 170:723–33.
10. Baldwin DS, Allgulander C, Bandelow B, Ferre F, Pallanti S: An international survey of reported prescribing practice in the treatment of patients with generalised anxiety disorder. World J Biol Psychiatry 2012; 13:510–16.
11. Offidani E, Guidi J, Tomba E, Fava GA: Efficacy and tolerability of benzodiazepines versus antidepressants in anxiety disorders. Psychother Psychosom 2013; 82:355–62.
12. Quagliato LA, Cosci F, Shader RI, Silbermann EK, Starcevic V, Balon R, Dubovsky SL, Salzman C, Krystal JH, Weintraub SJ, Freire RC, Nardi AE: Selective serotonin reuptake inhibitors and benzodiazepines in panic disorder. J Psychopharmacol 2019; 33:1340–51.
13. Chouinard G: Issues in the clinical use of benzodiazepines: potency, withdrawal and rebound. J Clin Psychiatry 2004; 65 (Suppl. 5):7–12.
14. Cosci F, Chouinard G: Acute and persistent withdrawal syndromes following discontinuation of psychotropic medications. Psychother Psychosom 2020; 89:283–306.
15. Benasi G, Guidi J, Offidani E, Balon R, Rickels K, Fava GA: Benzodiazepines as a monotherapy in depressive disorder. Psychother Psychosom 2018; 87:65–74.
16. Cloos JM, Bocquest V, Rolland-Portal I, Koch P, Chouinard G: Hypnotics and triazolobenzodiazepines—best predictors of high-dose benzodiazepine use. Psychother Psychosom 2015; 84:273–83.
17. Teboul E, Chouinard G: A guide to benzodiazepine selection. Part I: pharmacological aspects. Can J Psychiatry 1990; 35:700–10.
18. Clark DA, Beck AT: Cognitive Therapy of Anxiety Disorders. New York, Guilford, 2010.
19. Offidani E, Fava GA, Tomba E, Baldessarini RJ: Excessive mood elevation and behavioral activation with antidepressant treatment of juvenile depressive and anxiety disorders. Psychother Psychosom 2013; 82:132–41.
20. Richardson WS, Doster LM: Comorbidity and multimorbidity need to be placed in the context of a framework of risk, responsiveness, and vulnerability. J Clin Epidemiol 2014; 67:244–6.
21. Fava GA, Belaise C: Discontinuing antidepressants drugs. Lesson from a failed trial and extensive clinical experience. Psychother Psychosom 2018; 87:257–67.
22. Fava GA: Evidence-based medicine was bound to fail. J Clin Epidemiol 2017; 84:3–7.
23. Abramson J: Overdosed America. New York, Harper-Collins Publishers, 2005.
24. Fava M: Diagnosis and definition of treatment-resistant depression. Biol Psychiatry 2003; 53:649–59.
25. Fava GA, Cosci F, Guidi J, Rafanelli C: The deceptive manifestations of treatment resistance in depression. Psychother Psychosom 2020; 89:265–73.
26. Dubovsky SL: What is new about new antidepressants? Psychother Psychosom 2018; 87:129–39.

27. Dold M, Bartova L, Rupprecht R, Kasper S: Dose escalation of antidepressants in unipolar depression: a meta-analysis of double-blind, randomized controlled trials. Psychother Psychosom 2017; 86:283–91.
28. Bschor T, Kern H, Henssler J, Baethge C: Switching the antidepressant after nonresponse in adults with major depression: a systematic literature search and meta-analysis. J Clin Psychiatry 2018; 79(1):16r10749.
29. Cosci F, Fava GA: The clinical inadequacy of the DSM-5 classification of somatic symptoms and related disorders: an alternative trans-diagnostic model. CNS Spectrums 2016; 21:310–17.
30. de las Cuevas, de Leon J: Reviving research on medication attitudes for improving pharmacotherapy. Psychother Psychosom 2017; 86:73–9.
31. Di Mascio A: Personality and variability of response to psychotropic drugs: relationship to "paradoxical" effect. In: Rickels K (ed). Non-Specific Factors in Drug Therapy. Springfield, IL, Charles C. Thomas, 1968, pp. 40–9.
32. Guidi J, Fava GA: The emerging role of euthymia in psychotherapy research and practice. Clin Psychol Rev 2020; 82:101941.
33. Guidi J, Fava GA, Picardi A, Porcelli P, Bellomo, Grandi S, Grassi L, Pasquini P, Quartesan R, Rafanelli C, Rigatelli M, Sonino N: Subtyping depression in the medically ill by cluster analysis. J Affect Disord 2011; 132:383–8.
34. Fava GA, Guidi J, Rafanelli C, Rickels K: The clinical inadequacy of the placebo model and the development of an alternative conceptual framework. Psychother Psychosom 2017; 86:332–40.
35. Maund E, Stuart B, Moore M, Dowrick C, Geraghty AWA, Dawson S, Kendrick T: Managing antidepressant discontinuation. Ann Fam Med 2019; 17:52–60.
36. Keller MB, Lavori PW, Mueller TI, Endicott J, Coryell W, Hirschfeld RMA, Shea T: Time to recovery, chronicity, and levels of psychopathology in major depression. Arch Gen Psychiatry 1992; 49:809–16.
37. Guidi J, Tomba E, Fava GA: The sequential integration of pharmacotherapy and psychotherapy in the treatment of major depressive disorder: a meta-analysis of the sequential model and a critical review of the literature. Am J Psychiatry 2016; 173:128–37.
38. Guidi J, Fava GA: Sequential combination of pharmacotherapy and psychotherapy in major depressive disorder: a systematic review and meta-analysis. JAMA Psychiatry 2021; 78:261-9.
39. Cosci F, Mansueto G, Fava GA: Relapse prevention in recurrent major depressive disorder. Int J Psychiatry Clin Pract 2020; 24:341–8.
40. Fava GA, Tomba E: New modalities of assessment and treatment planning in depression. The sequential approach. CNS Drugs 2010; 24:453–65.
41. Menza M, Marin H, Sokol Opper R: Residual symptoms in depression: can treatment be symptom-specific? J Clin Psychiatr 2003; 64:516–23.
42. Bilsker D, Wiseman S, Gilbert M: Managing depression-related occupational disability. Can J Psychiatry 2006; 51:76–83.
43. Kennedy N, Foy K, Sherazi R, McDonough M, McKean P: Long-term social functioning after depression treated by psychiatrists. Bipolar Disord 2007; 9:25–37.
44. Chuang HT, Mansell C, Patten SB: Lifestyle characteristics of psychiatric outpatients. Can J Psychiatry 2008; 53:260–6.

45. Judd LJ, Paulus MJ, Schettler PJ, Akiskal HS, Endicott J, Leon AC, Maser JD, Mueller T, Solomon DA, Keller MB: Does incomplete recovery from first lifetime major depressive episode herald a chronic course of illness? Am J Psychiatry 2000; 157:1501–4.
46. Fava GA: The hidden costs of financial conflicts of interest in medicine. Psychother Psychosom 2016; 85:65–70.

13

A Different Psychiatry Is Possible

Part of the challenge and, at the same time, fascination of being a clinician lies in applying the scientific method to the care of individual patients (1). Increased knowledge would result in significant benefits for the patients and in a sense of continued development for the physician. Probably no other professional would look at the literature with the same interest and expectations as a clinician. A researcher, not involved in clinical care, is primarily concerned with his/her specific, and usually quite narrow, area. A clinician, however, has to face the highly heterogeneous and complex domains of clinical encounters. Yet, this pathway seems to be getting more and more difficult, regardless of the specialty of the physician (2). The fact that clinicians may no longer find any journal articles relevant to their practice is a serious problem and a source of frustration. "Are we getting old and no longer have enough time and patience for keeping up with the literature?". "Has research become too complicated?" (2). These are explanations that clinicians may find to justify their progressive detachment from research. At times, these questions are accompanied by a sense of personal stagnation and tiredness, which makes clinical duties less tolerable in health systems that are more and more characterized by the eclipse of humane relationships (2).

These feelings pervade all areas of medicine, but are particularly pronounced in psychiatry. In the past two decades, an increasing number of psychiatrists, from all over the country, have requested a consultation with me for personal problems such as depressed mood, burn-out, and insomnia. A common theme has been that the hope that clinical problems in psychiatry could be ultimately solved by the progress made in the neurosciences, and especially in psychopharmacology, has evaporated. The cures and insights that the neurosciences had promised have not taken place. Indeed, the profession appears to be facing more difficulties and challenges. Is this due to more demanding environmental circumstances or to something else? Once again, Alvan Feinstein (3) had anticipated such a crisis and attributed it to the decline of clinical medicine as the source of fundamental scientific challenges, which took place after the Second World War: "The preclinical sciences became detached from their clinical origins and were converted into 'basic biomedical sciences' with goals that often no longer aimed at mechanisms of disease, with investigators who often had no clinical training or responsibilities, and with results that often had no overt relationship to clinical phenomena" (3, p.216). The consequences were probably more severe in psychiatry than in any other medical discipline and yielded a major crisis, which I will discuss. However, such a crisis can be overcome and may lead to a redefinition of the discipline and its approach.

The Crisis of Psychiatry as a Medical Discipline

In a paper published in a leading psychiatric journal (4), Heinz Katschnig wondered whether psychiatrists are an endangered species: the validity of classification systems is increasingly questioned; confidence in the results of therapeutic interventions is waning; psychiatry has a low status within medicine and the society in general, and its field of competence is increasingly threatened by other professions; and the recruitment into psychiatry is declining. I have attributed the main causes of this decline to an intellectual crisis (2), which articulates over several converging trends, outlined below.

Loss of Clinical Practice as a Source
of Scientific Investigation

Research has become more and more detached from clinical challenges. The neurosciences have exported their conceptual framework into psychiatry much more than serving as an investigative tool for addressing the questions raised by clinical practice. In the previous chapters, I have given several examples of common and vexing problems, such as withdrawal reactions and loss of clinical efficacy, that have not received adequate research attention. There is clearly a missing link between bio-markers and clinical states in mental disorders (5).

Biological Reductionism

It is the tendency to view complex clinical phenomena as ultimately de-rived from a single primary cause (e.g., genetic) instead of using a mul-tifactorial frame of reference (6). Biological reductionism has resulted in an idealistic approach, which is quite far from the explanatory pluralism required by clinical practice (7). This applies to both the methodology of clinical trials and the clinician's approach. If a physician disregards the importance of non-drug contributions and does not spend time with the patient for improving such contributions, then the limitations of isolated, magic-bullet interventions (whether medications or psychotherapy) are likely to emerge (8). An important drive to reductionism has been the growth of EBM, which is likely to concentrate on single factors, and fail to give suitable weight to clinical variables and the incremental value of single therapeutic components (9).

Limitations of Diagnostic Criteria

The introduction of diagnostic criteria for the identification of psychi-atric syndromes has considerably decreased the variance due to different assessors and the use of inferential criteria rather than direct observa-tion. There is, however, increasing awareness of the limitations of the current diagnostic systems (10, 11). Very seldom, comorbid diagnoses undergo hierarchical organization or attention is paid to the longitu-dinal development of mental illnesses (e.g., staging) (10). Exclusive re-liance on diagnostic criteria has impoverished the clinical process and does not reflect the complex thinking that underlies decisions in psy-chiatric practice (10). An initial cross-sectional examination with a very narrow focus seems to generate a number of "automatic" decisions, as a result of algorithms or guidelines, with few opportunities for modifying the initial judgment.

Detachment of Research from Clinical Needs

A good deal of research funds are unable to address basic clinical questions and exclude most of the RCTs (that are generally done by and for the benefit of the industry). The phenomenon is particularly pronounced in the United States, with the emphasis on biological markers (12) and psychopathology (the analysis of signs and symptoms in psychiatry) and clinical judgment discarded as non-scientific and obsolete methods. The futility of looking for pretreatment biological predictors to find clinical solutions for the entire course of illness is obvious, since neurobiological assets change throughout the course of the disorder and recovery is a one-way street which does not lead back to the premorbid condition, as described in Chapter 4.

Psychiatric Versus Non-Specialist Interventions

The intellectual crisis of psychiatric research (2, 4) has major reflections on clinical practice. A number of studies had indicated the failure of mental health specialists to improve the outcome of depression in the primary care setting. Simon et al. (13) compared the 6-month outcome in depressed patients receiving antidepressant prescriptions either from psychiatrists or from primary care physicians. The two groups showed similar rates of improvement in all measures of symptom severity and functioning. Similar results were obtained with the collaboration of primary care physicians and mental health consultants (14), implementation of clinical practice guidelines (15), and randomization to a relapse prevention programme or usual primary care (16). The findings indicate that the average depressed patient has no better chance of getting and remaining well with the psychiatric specialist than with his/her primary care physician. This is in sharp contrast with the expectations that non-psychiatric physicians may have and is one of the explanations for the exclusion of psychiatrists from primary care approaches to depression and anxiety (17). Not surprisingly, also, the indications emerging from mainstream psychiatry for managing withdrawal syndromes (essentially going back to the same or a similar antidepressant) are clearly inadequate (see Chapter 8), and psychiatrists are excluded or have a very marginal role in national health service efforts to address the problem (18).

The Growing Influence of the Pharmaceutical Industry

Psychiatry is affected by the contamination of conflict of interest as much as any other medical specialty (2). Corporate actions have affected the shaping of guidelines, placed undue expectations on new medications, and provided misleading indications to the practicing psychiatrists. Iatrogenic effects have been hidden from clinical attention, such as in the case of withdrawal syndromes from discontinuing antidepressant drugs.

However, the approach that has been described in this book departs from conventional ways of evaluating and treating depression, as well as other psychiatric disturbances. The assessment, management, and prevention strategies I suggest follow a different type of psychiatry, which is worth examining.

Guide to a Clinical Revolution: Key Issues for a Renewed Foundation of Psychiatric Practice

Broadening the Targets of the Assessment

Formulating a diagnosis according to diagnostic criteria is a necessary but quite insufficient step for an adequate assessment (10). With the use of clinimetrics, we may expand the targets of the evaluation to issues such as the patient's environment and illness behavior (see Chapter 7). Further, the longitudinal development of disorders and comorbidities may also be considered according to staging methods (10).

Thinking "Iatrogenic"

The iatrogenic perspective—the fact that a treatment a patient received or is currently receiving (whether pharmacotherapy or psychotherapy) may play a causative role in part of the symptomatology—has been banned from clinical thinking, as a dangerous anti-psychiatry element, while it is essential with the increasing use of psychotropic medications and/or psychotherapies (19). The traditional treatment and medication history should include tracking of medication discontinuation, withdrawal symptomatology, and other forms of behavioral toxicity, as detailed in Chapter 3. Exploring the hypothesis of persistent postwithdrawal disorders may shed some light on a variety of clinical manifestations (19). Currently, clinicians are mostly unable to formulate tentative hypotheses, to be verified by further assessment, in iatrogenic terms (19).

The Many Forms of Comorbidity and the Unifying Framework of Macroanalysis

Limiting the concept of comorbidity to the co-occurrence of other psychiatric disorders is a substantial weakness of the current approach and is at variance with other medical specialties (10). There are many issues that may play a role in the persistence of disturbances, from the psychosocial environment to iatrogenic comorbidity. Some elements that may be therapeutic in most patients may prove anti-therapeutic for other individuals (see Chapter 12). Macroanalysis offers an opportunity for an operational framework, where priorities and relationships can be established (see Chapter 7).

Repeated Assessments

Repeated assessments are the mainstay of the sequential model (20). If properly performed (not just medication checks), they not only allow for the monitoring of the patient's progress but may also disclose psychopathological elements that are overshadowed by the acute manifestations of the disorder. Moreover, with increasingly complicated cases, a single initial evaluation may not be sufficient for satisfactory assessment and treatment planning. A second evaluation (2–3 weeks later) may disclose important information about the course of the disorder, may offer the opportunity to get important data that the patient forgot to report and/or to involve significant others, and takes advantage of the use of the patient's diary as an additional source of clinimetric information (21).

Diagnoses as Transfer Stations

Tinetti and Fried (22) argued that the time has come to abandon disease as the focus of medical care—and a similar consideration may
apply to psychiatric disorders. Today, the changed spectrum of health
conditions (e.g., multimorbidity, chronicity) points to the inadequa-
cies of medical care that is centered primarily on the diagnosis and
treatment of each disease separately (22). Clinical decision-making,
for all patients, should address the attainment of individual goals and
the identification and treatment of all modifiable and non- biological
factors, rather than focus solely on the diagnosis and treatment of individual diseases (22). Similar considerations pertain to psychiatric
diseases (10). Identification of disorders thus takes the form of "transfer
stations" (23) that are amenable to longitudinal verification and modification as long as therapeutic goals are achieved. A DSM diagnosis is just
the beginning of the diagnostic process; it is a necessary but insufficient
step in evaluation.

Individualized Focus of Therapy

The American Psychiatric Association guideline for the treatment of patients with major depressive disorder states:

> The ultimate recommendation regarding a particular clinical proce-
> dure or treatment plan must be made by the psychiatrist in light of the
> clinical data, the psychiatric evaluation, and the diagnostic and treat-
> ment options available. Such recommendations should incorporate the
> patient's personal and socio-cultural preferences and values in order
> to enhance the therapeutic alliance, adherence to treatment, and treat-
> ment outcomes. (24, p.9)

However, guidance on how to implement this into operational actions
is missing, and identification of a disorder translates into an automatic
treatment option (10). Clinical decisions concerned with the application of knowledge to the individual patient need to be filtered by clinical
judgment and placed in the framework of potential benefits, likelihood of
responsiveness to the treatment option, and vulnerability to the adverse

effects of therapy (25). This latter point is particularly important in view of the increasing awareness of adverse events linked to antidepressant therapy (see Chapters 2–4). In the sequential model, therapeutic targets cannot be predetermined, but depend on the response of patients to the first course of treatment. Indeed, it is wishful thinking to believe that one course of treatment, whatever it may be, is sufficient to yield enduring remission in most of the clinical cases that are encountered today (10).

Targets of Treatment Interventions

The psychiatric paradigm still endorses the conviction that psychotropic drugs or psychotherapies "cure" diseases, while they actually address some aspects of the disorder (10). Moncrieff and Cohen (26) advocated a model of understanding the action of psychotropic drugs that would place more emphasis on subjective experience, develop outcome measures addressing particular behaviors rather than disorders, overcome the distinction between therapeutic and adverse effects, and evaluate patients' comparative preferences for different types of drugs in various situations. Similarly, Isaac Marks (27) underscored how psychotherapeutic treatments should be geared to improving problems reliably and enduringly, and pointed out the importance of understanding why psychotherapy components help only some sufferers and not others with the same problem. The pursuit of euthymia can no longer be ignored as a target of treatment (28). It should be conceived as a transdiagnostic strategy to be incorporated in individualized therapeutic plans. Psychotherapeutic techniques, such as WBT, should follow clinical reasoning and case formulation facilitated by the use of macroanalysis and staging. In a sequential treatment plan, therapeutic interventions (whether pharmacotherapy or psychotherapy) should be selected based on clinical judgment, taking into consideration a number of clinical variables, such as characteristics and severity of the psychiatric episode, co-occurring symptomatology and problems (not necessarily syndromes), iatrogenic factors, medical comorbidities, patient's history, and preferences (28).

Multidisciplinary Treatment Team

In clinical medicine, the traditional boundaries between medical specialties, based mostly on organ systems (e.g., cardiology, gastroenterology), appear to be more and more inadequate in dealing with symptoms and problems that require an integrated approach (29). Psychiatry makes no exception. In Chapter 6, I describe a multidisciplinary treatment team, which consists of a psychiatrist (with adequate background knowledge both in psychopharmacology and psychotherapy), an internist, and clinical psychotherapists, who may provide evidence-based treatments after the initial evaluation of the psychiatrist. Its functioning emphasizes joint assessments, sequential combination of treatments, and close coordination of team members, in line with emerging trends in mental healthcare delivery (30).

All these features strongly reflect the psychosomatic approach (29) and a reappraisal of the role of clinical judgment (10). An issue that is generally neglected in today's climate characterized by EBM is the fact that, when transferred to clinical medicine from their origin in agricultural research, RCTs were not intended to answer questions about the treatment of individual patients (31). There is no simple "average" solution to most medical problems. The question is how to put the available evidence within the context of individual, unique assets and liabilities. There is thus the need of integrating the information that derives from EBM with medicine-based evidence (MBE). Every physician has a personal library of clinical experiences (32), as this book exemplifies. Such experiences can be shared with the creation of database profiles where one can match the patient at hand (33). MBE can provide fundamental insights about the features, prognosis, and long-term outcomes of disturbances such as persistent postwithdrawal disorders. We desperately need the type of investigation that is at risk of disappearing from journals: naturalistic studies of psychiatric populations according to clinimetric and neurobiologic profiles. Further, the sequential model design allows patients who are already in treatment to be randomized and assigned to treatment alternatives according to stages of illness development and individual history, and not simply to disease classification. As a result, its implementation in research on depression may help in developing therapeutic strategies that are concerned with the patient population of everyday practice (20).

One can object that the approach described in this section and the rest of the book is unrealistic and requires an abrupt change from current practice. However, in their everyday work, psychiatrists use observation, description, and classification, test explanatory hypotheses, and formulate clinical decisions. In evaluating whether a patient needs admission to the hospital (or can be discharged from it), in deciding whether a patient needs treatment (and in that case, what type), and in planning the schedule of follow-up visits or interventions, the psychiatrist uses nothing more than the science of psychopathology and clinical judgment (10). The following case illustrates how the approach can be implemented by any psychiatrist in public and private practice.

Case Illustration

Roberta is a 64-year-old married woman who is referred to me by her primary care physician as a case of "resistant depression"; she has no previous history of mood or anxiety disturbances. I try to get to know some biographical background first, with open-ended questions. She had been working all her life in a bakery with her husband, raising two children. A couple of years ago, she and her husband received a good offer to sell the bakery; her husband was strongly in favor (the job was very tough, even though he liked it; getting up so early every morning to prepare and bake the bread was increasingly tiring). So they sold their bakery and retired, with many projects in mind, including spending more time with their grandchildren.

However, Roberta progressively felt more and more anxious, tense, and irritable. She started having trouble falling asleep and, at a later point in time, she was also waking up early without being able to go back to sleep. Her motivation decreased and she spent more and more time at home, avoiding any social and family contact, including with the grandchildren. She went to her primary care physician who diagnosed a depressive state and prescribed sertraline (50 mg/day). Since there was little effect after a month, her doctor increased sertraline to 100 mg/day. This time a clear effect ensued: nausea and stomach burning. She asked her doctor, "Isn't it this medication that is causing all this? I never had them before." The doctor was reassuring: "Absolutely not. These are not side effects of this medication." When she told me this, I thought, "The spectacular achievements of propaganda. These are very common side effects." Her doctor added: "It is the stress that is causing all this. In any event, I am changing the antidepressant to something stronger." He prescribed venlafaxine: first 75 mg/day, then 150 mg/day. He also prescribed anti-nausea medications and protein pump inhibitors. Yet, nausea persisted.

Since venlafaxine had failed to yield clinical improvement, Roberta's physician referred her to our service "for psychotherapy." I started enquiring about specific symptoms. Roberta had indeed a major depressive disorder, associated with ruminations and avoidance, which approached the threshold of agoraphobia. Her refusals to go out created tension with her husband. A very important issue to explore is how the patients spend their days, and their lifestyle. She was mostly at home, missing the bakery and the good old times. She was also worried about her stomach problems and was afraid of something bad on the way ("I heard of so many people who got cancer when they retired").

The macroanalysis then takes the form depicted in Figure 13.1. It illustrates the links between various components and how they reinforce each other in a vicious cycle. First of all, I told her that the nausea and gastric burning were probably related to the medication (she was angry and

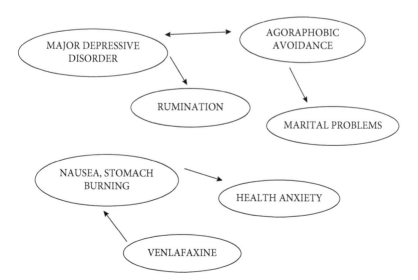

Figure 13.1 Baseline Assessment According to Macroanalysis

wondered why her doctor had denied it). "It is not your doctor's fault," I tried to say. "The pharmaceutical industries do not let the doctors know about many side effects." (I did not want to spoil her relationship with him.) "I am going to change your antidepressant with another that has a protective action on your stomach and that is going to help you get better," I informed her. I chose mirtazapine, 15 mg/day. "The medication you are taking (venlafaxine) is likely to cause some problems when I discontinue it." (She had indeed had some new withdrawal symptoms when switching from sertraline to venlafaxine.) "Do you prefer a rapid switch, which is likely to cause more problems, or a gradual one?" She was emphatic: "For God's sake, get this rubbish out of my body as soon as possible." I did: I changed venlafaxine abruptly for mirtazapine, with no intermediate step, warning her of some likely problems in the first 2 weeks. I added, however, that the medication I was prescribing would contribute, at best, 50% to her getting better. (I know, in reality, it is likely to be less, but I try to convey a little optimism.) I wrote out another prescription for "self-therapy" (Box 13.1), emphasizing that what I was asking her to do would contribute to the other 50% of getting better. I kept her on the anti-nausea medication and the protein pump inhibitors for the time being. Roberta had to call me in a week to tell me how it was going, and I scheduled to see her in a month. The macroanalysis (Figure 13.2) now reflects my intervention, consisting of an appropriate medication, explanatory therapy, and homework exposure.

She called after a week. She had indeed experienced some withdrawal symptoms, but had a strong motivation to endure ("my stomach is saying thanks"). When I saw her after a month, she was definitely improved in

---

Box 13.1 Roberta's Self-Therapy

- Go out every morning alone for 5–10 minutes.
- Go out every afternoon with your husband and walk for at least half an hour.
- Report what you do in a diary.
- Refrain from staying inactive in the house.
- Visit your grandchildren twice per week.

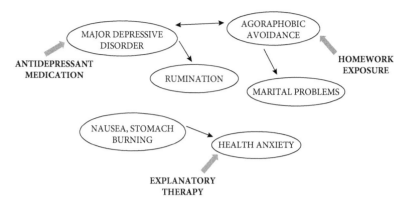

Figure 13.2 Therapeutic Targets According to Macroanalysis

terms of sleep, mood, and energy, yet she still spent most of her days at home ruminating. Her nausea and stomach burning were almost gone, and she was very pleased about that. I then challenged her: "We are doing better, but not well. We now have two choices: one is to increase the medication to 30 mg of mirtazapine per day; the other is that you work more on your tasks." Roberta replied: "You put your 50%, I am positive; I put 10 or 20% of mine at best. It is my turn: I must increase my efforts. Let us keep the medication the way it is. I have your second prescription. I just need to follow it better." I emphasized again the importance of self-therapy and I let her know that, if needed, there was a psychologist in my group who could help her with it. "But let us see what you do now." After another month, she had definitely improved in all areas. She was going out with her husband, planning a little trip, and visiting her grandchildren. "Both prescriptions were necessary," she commented. "What about the other medications?" she asked. I replied: "I would like a colleague of mine in our group, an internist, to have a look at you and to decide. She may also check your general physical health." (I know that our internist's full physical examination is worth more than all our reassuring words.) "We'll now see you in 3 months, unless something happens and you call me up." She wondered how long she would have to take mirtazapine. "We'll see then. If you continue to work with self-therapy and make even further progress, we may discontinue it. If you slow down, we may even have to increase it." After 3 months she had further improved, and mirtazapine was stopped without tapering (because of the low dose); the other medications for nausea and stomach burning were discontinued as well. At a 4-year follow-up, the patient was well and drug-free.

The management of this patient involved a total of four psychiatric visits (45 minutes each) and one consultation with the internist. The case illustrates how attention to the patient narrative (biography) is the neglected basic method in the care of patients (33), and how macroanalysis helps in formulating an individualized treatment plan. It underscores the value of including iatrogenic effects in the evaluation and the important role of psychotherapeutic management (not psychotherapy), in terms of explanatory therapy and homework exposure.

Conclusions

If we look at the major health problems caused by inappropriate prescriptions of antidepressant medications, at the fact that we have so little scientific information to deal with key clinical issues (such as those related to behavioral toxicity), and at the highly disappointing results of newer medications, we may become convinced that this is the worst of times for psychiatry. Clinical assessment in psychiatry is currently viewed as a historic relic, to be substituted by biomarkers and neuroscience methods (12). When? Ten, twenty years from now?

In the words of Charles Dickens, however, it may also be the best of times. Adequate evaluation of iatrogenic factors calls for a renaissance of psychopathology (observation, interviewing, classification and differential diagnosis of signs and symptoms) as the basic neglected method of clinical psychiatry (34). This may lead to overdue critical scrutiny of current conceptual models that clash with clinical reality. Psychiatrists, who in their clinical practice use sophisticated forms of clinical judgment and master techniques of interviewing and history taking, are ready to reveille something that has not vanished but is simply buried under irrelevant research, meta-junk, and inadequate conceptual models.

There are entire areas of clinical research—such as those related to the iatrogenic effects of medications and psychotherapy—that are largely unexplored and should become the preferred channel of funding and attention. Neuroscientific methods applied to circumscribed problems (e.g., what actually characterizes withdrawal syndromes) may offer unprecedented opportunities but should be associated with clinimetric tools (e.g., specific criteria). Unlike psychopharmacology, psychotherapy has made major advances in the past two decades, and even greater progress may take place if proper funding for research and full inclusion in the national health service are assured.

Psychiatrists have the potential to move from the traditionally assigned position as marginal components of the medical profession (35) to leaders in multidisciplinary medicine and in an overdue reappraisal of EBM (2, 8), in favor of the role of clinical judgment (10).

Personalized/precision medicine, referred to as genomics-based knowledge, promises to approach each patient as the biological individual he/she is (36). However, the practical applications have still a long way to go, and neglect of psychological and social features may actually lead to "depersonalized" medicine (33, 36). It is possible to practice highly effective precision psychiatry now, without waiting 10 to 20 years. For overcoming the problems related to the discontinuation of antidepressant medications, we have no other way.

References

1. Engel GL: Physician-scientists and scientific physicians. Am J Med 1987; 82:107–11.
2. Fava GA: The intellectual crisis of psychiatric research. Psychother Psychosom 2006; 75:202–8.
3. Feinstein AR: The intellectual crisis in clinical science. Persp Biol Med 1987; 30:215–30.
4. Katschnig H: Are psychiatrists an endangered species? World Psychiatry 2010; 9:21–8.
5. Fava GA, Guidi J, Grandi S, Hasler G: The missing link between clinical states and biomarkers in mental disorders. Psychother Psychosom 2014; 83:136–41.
6. Engel GL: The need for a new medical model: a challenge for biomedicine. Science 1977; 196:129–36.
7. Kendler KS: Toward a philosophical structure for psychiatry. Am J Psychiatry 2005; 162:433–40.
8. Fava GA, Sonino N: From the lesson of George Engel to current knowledge: the biopsychosocial model—40 years later. Psychother Psychosom 2017; 86:257–9.
9. Fava GA: Evidence-based medicine was bound to fail. J Clin Epidemiol 2017; 84:3–7.

10. Fava GA, Rafanelli C, Tomba E: The clinical process in psychiatry: a clinimetric approach. J Clin Psychiatry 2012; 73:177–84.
11. Thombs BD, Turner KA, Shrier I: Defining and evaluating overdiagnosis in mental health. Psychother Psychosom 2019; 88:193–202.
12. Cuthbert BN: The RDoC framework: facilitating transition from ICD-DSM to dimensional approaches that integrate neuroscience and psychopathology. World Psychiatry 2014; 13:28–35.
13. Simon GE, Von Korff M, Rutter CM, Peterson DA: Treatment process and outcomes for managed care patients receiving new antidepressant prescriptions from psychiatrists and primary care physicians. Arch Gen Psychiatry 2001; 58:395–401.
14. Lin EHB, Simon GE, Katon WJ, Russo JE, Von Korff M, Bush TM, Ludman EJ, Walker EA: Can enhanced acute-phase treatment of depression improve long-term outcomes? Am J Psychiatry 1999; 156:643–5.
15. Thompson C, Kinmonth AL, Stevens L, Peveler RC, Stevens A, Ostler KJ, Pickering RM, Baker NG, Henson A, Preece J, Cooper D, Campbell MJ: Effects of a clinical practice guideline and practice-based education on detection and outcome of depression in primary care. Lancet 2000; 355:185–91.
16. Katon WJ, Rutter C, Ludman EJ, Von Korff M, Lin E, Simon G, Bush T, Walker E, Unutzer J: A randomized trial of relapse prevention of depression in primary care. Arch Gen Psychiatry 2001; 58:241–7.
17. Layard R: The case for psychological treatment centres. BMJ 2006; 332:1030–2.
18. Kendrick T: Strategies to reduce use of antidepressants. Br J Clin Pharmacol 2021; 87:23–33.
19. Fava GA, Rafanelli C: Iatrogenic factors in psychopathology. Psychother Psychosom 2019; 88:129–40.
20. Fava GA, Tomba E: New modalities of assessment and treatment planning in depression. The sequential approach. CNS Drugs 2010; 24:453–65.
21. Guidi J, Fava GA: The emerging role of euthymia in psychotherapy research and practice. Clin Psychol Rev 2020; 82:101941.
22. Tinetti ME, Fried T: The end of the disease era. Am J Med 2004; 116:179–85.
23. Feinstein AR: An analysis of diagnostic reasoning. I: The domains and disorders of clinical macrobiology. Yale J Biol Med 1973; 46:212–32.
24. American Psychiatric Association: Practice guideline for the treatment of patients with major depressive disorder. Third edition. Am J Psychiatry 2010; 167 (Suppl.):1–118.
25. Richardson WS, Doster LM: Comorbidity and multimorbidity need to be placed in the context of a framework of risk, responsiveness, and vulnerability. J Clin Epidemiol 2014; 67:244–6.
26. Moncrieff J, Cohen D: Rethinking models of psychotropic drug action. Psychother Psychosom 2005; 74:145–53.
27. Marks IM: The maturing of therapy. Br J Psychiatry 2002; 180:200–4.
28. Fava GA, Guidi J: The pursuit of euthymia. World Psychiatry 2020; 19:40–50.
29. Fava GA, Cosci F, Sonino N: Current psychosomatic practice. Psychother Psychosom 2017; 86:13–30.
30. Marks I: Mental health clinics in the 21st century. Psychother Psychosom 2009; 78:133–8.

31. Feinstein AR, Horwitz RI: Problems in the 'evidence' of 'evidence-based medicine'. Am J Med 1997; 103:529–35.
32. Feinstein AR, Rubinstein JF, Ramshaw WA: Estimating prognosis with the aid of conversational-mode computer program. Ann Intern Med 1972; 911–21.
33. Lobitz G, Armstrong K, Concato J, Singer BH, Horwitz RI: The biological and biographical basis of precision medicine. Psychother Psychosom 2019; 88:333–40.
34. Lipowski ZJ: Psychopathology as a science: its scope and tasks. Compr Psychiatry 1966; 7:175–82.
35. Smith HL: Psychiatry in medicine: intra- or inter-professional relationships? Am J Sociol 1957; 63:285–9.
36. Horwitz RI, Cullen MR, Abell J, Christian JB: (De)personalized medicine. Science 2012; 339:1155–6.

Index

For the benefit of digital users, indexed terms that span two pages (e.g., 52–53) may, on occasion, appear on only one of those pages.

Tables, figures and boxes are indicated by *t*, *f* and *b* following the page number